KARMA - YOGA

THE YOGA OF ACTION

Sumanth Batchu

SWAMI VIVEKANANDA

CONGRATULATIONS!

TED Talk-2015

Vidya-Niketanam

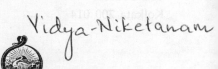

Advaita Ashrama

(PUBLICATION DEPARTMENT)

5 DEHI ENTALLY ROAD · KOLKATA 700 014

Published by
Swami Bodhasarananda
Adhyaksha, Advaita Ashrama
Mayavati, Champawat, Uttarakhand, Himalayas
from its Publication Department, Kolkata
Email: mail@advaitaashrama.org
Website: www.advaitaashrama.org

Forty-sixth Reprint, August 2013
5M3C

ISBN 978-81-85301-89-1

Printed in India at
Trio Process
Kolkata 700 014

CONTENTS

CONTENTS

KARMA IN ITS EFFECT ON CHARACTER

THE word Karma is derived from the Sanskrit Kri, to do; all action is Karma. Technically, this word also means the effects of actions. In connection with metaphysics, it sometimes means the effects, of which our past actions were the causes. But in Karma-Yoga we have simply to do with the word Karma as meaning work. The goal of mankind is knowledge. That is the one ideal placed before us by Eastern philosophy. Pleasure is not the goal of man, but knowledge. Pleasure and happiness come to an end. It is a mistake to suppose that pleasure is the goal. The cause of all the miseries we have in the world is that men foolishly think pleasure to be the ideal to strive for. After a time man finds that it is not happiness, but knowledge, towards which he is going, and that both pleasure and pain are great teachers; and that he learns as much from evil as from good. As pleasure and pain pass before his soul, they leave upon it different pictures, and the result of these combined impressions is what is called man's "character". If you take the character of any man, it really is but the aggregate of tendencies, the sum total of the bent of his mind; you will find that misery and happiness are equal factors in the formation of that character. Good and evil have an equal share in moulding character, and in some instances misery is a greater teacher than happiness. In studying the great characters the world has produced, I dare say, in the vast majority of cases it would be found that it was misery that taught more than happiness, it was poverty that taught more than wealth, it was blows that brought out their inner fire more than praise.

Now this knowledge, again, is inherent in man. No knowledge comes from outside; it is all inside. What we say a man "knows", should, in strict psychological language, be what he "discovers" or "unveils", what a man "learns" is really what he "discovers", by taking the cover off his own soul, which is a mine of infinite knowledge. We say Newton discovered gravitation. Was it sitting anywhere in a corner waiting for him? It was in his own mind; the time came and he found it out. All knowledge that the world has ever received comes from the mind; the infinite library of the universe is in your own mind. The external world is simply the suggestion, the occasion, which sets you to study your own mind, but the object of your study is always your own mind. The falling of an apple gave the suggestion to Newton, and he studied his own mind. He rearranged all the previous links of thought in his mind and discovered a new link among them, which we call the law of gravitation. It was not in the apple nor in anything in the centre of the earth. All knowledge, therefore, secular or spiritual, is in the human mind. In many cases it is not discovered but remains covered, and when the covering is being slowly taken off we say, "We are learning", and the advance of knowledge is made by the advance of this process of uncovering. The man from whom this veil is being lifted is the more knowing man; the man upon whom it lies thick is ignorant; and the man from whom it has entirely gone is all-knowing, omniscient. There have been omniscient men, and, I believe, there will be yet; and that there will be myriads of them in the cycles to come. Like fire in a piece of flint, knowledge exists in the mind; suggestion is the friction which brings it out. So with all our feelings and actions—our tears and our smiles, our joys and our griefs, our weeping and our laughter, our curses and our blessings, our praises and our blames—every one of these we may find, if we calmly study our own selves, to have been brought out from within ourselves by so many blows. The result is what we are. All these blows taken together are called Karma—work, action. Every mental and physical blow that is given to the soul, by which, as it were, fire is struck from it, and by which its own power and knowledge are discovered, is Karma, this word being used in its widest sense; thus we are all doing Karma all the time. I am talking to you: that is Karma. You are listening: that is Karma. We breathe: that is Karma. We walk: Karma. Everything we do, physical or mental, is Karma, and it leaves its marks on us.

There are certain works which are, as it were, the aggregate, the sum total, of a large number of smaller works. If we stand near the seashore and hear the waves dashing against the shingle, we think it is such a great noise; and yet we know that one wave is really composed of millions and millions of minute waves. Each one of these is making a noise, and yet we do not catch it; it is only when they become the big aggregate that we hear. Similarly, every pulsation of the heart is work; certain kinds of work we feel and they become tangible to us; they are, at the same time, the aggregate of a number of small works. If you really want to judge of the character of a man, look not at his great performances. Every fool may become a hero at one time or another. Watch a man do his most common actions; those are indeed the things which will tell you the real character of a great man. Great occasions rouse even the lowest of human beings to some kind of greatness, but he alone is the really great man whose character is great always, the same wherever he be.

Karma in its effect on character is the most tremendous power that man has to deal with. Man is, as it were, a centre, and is attracting all the powers of the universe towards himself, and in this centre is fusing them all and again sending them off in a big current. Such a centre is the *real* man, the almighty, the omniscient, and he draws the whole universe towards him. Good and bad, misery and happiness, all are running towards him and clinging round him; and out of them he fashions the mighty stream of tendency called character and throws it outwards. As he has the power of drawing in anything, so has he the power of throwing it out.

All the actions that we see in the world, all the movements in human society, all the works that we have around us, are simply the display of thought, the manifestation of the will of man. Machines or instruments, cities, ships or men-of-war, all these are simply the manifestation of the will of man; and this will is caused by character and character is manufactured by Karma. As is Karma, so is the manifestation of the will. The men of mighty will the world has produced have all been tremendous workers— gigantic souls with wills powerful enough to overturn worlds, wills they got by persistent work through ages and ages. Such a gigantic will as that of a Buddha or a Jesus could not be obtained in one life, for we know who their fathers were. It is not known that their fathers ever spoke a word for the good of mankind. Millions and millions of carpenters like Joseph had gone; millions are still living. Millions and millions of petty kings like Buddha's father had been in the world. If it was only a case of hereditary transmission, how do you account for this petty prince who was not, perhaps, obeyed by his own servants, producing this son whom half a world worships? How do you explain the gulf between the carpenter and his son whom millions of human beings worship as God? It cannot be solved by the theory of heredity. The gigantic will which Buddha and Jesus threw over the world, whence did it come? Whence came this accumulation of power? It must have been there through ages and ages, continually growing bigger and bigger, until it burst on society in a Buddha or a Jesus, even rolling down to the present day.

All this is determined by Karma, work. No one can get anything unless he earns it; this is an eternal law. We may sometimes think it is not so, but in the long run we become convinced of it. A man may struggle all his life for riches; he may cheat thousands, but he finds at last that he did not deserve to become rich, and his life becomes a trouble and a nuisance to him. We may go on accumulating things for our physical enjoyment, but only what we earn is really ours. A fool may buy all the books in the world, and they will be in his library, but he will be able to read only those that he deserves to; and this deserving is produced by Karma. Our Karma determines what we deserve and what we can assimilate. We are responsible for what we are; and whatever we wish ourselves to be, we have the power to make ourselves. If what we are now has been the result of our own past actions, it certainly follows that whatever we wish to be in future can be produced by our present actions; so we have to know how to act. You will say, "What is the use of learning how to work? Everyone works in some way or other in this world." But there is such a thing as frittering away our energies. With regard to Karma-Yoga, the Gita says that it is doing work with cleverness and as a science: by knowing how to work, one can obtain the greatest results. You must remember that all work is simply to bring out the power of the mind which is already there, to wake up the soul. The power is inside every man, so is knowledge; the different works are like blows to bring them out, to cause these giants to wake up.

Man works with various motives; there cannot be work without motive. Some people want to get fame, and they work for fame. Others want money, and they work for money. Others want to have power, and they work for power. Others want to get to heaven, and they work for the same. Others want to leave a name when they die, as they do in China where no man gets a title until he is dead; and that is a better way, after all, than with us. When a man does something very good there, they give a title of nobility to his father who is dead, or to his grandfather. Some people work for that. Some of the followers of certain Mohammedan sects work all their lives to have a big tomb built for them when they die. I know sects among whom, as soon as a child is born, a tomb is prepared for it; that is among them the most important work a man has to do, and the bigger and the finer the tomb, the better off the man is supposed to be. Others work as a penance; do all sorts of wicked things, then erect a temple, or give something to the priests to buy them off and obtain from them a passport to heaven. They think that this kind of beneficence will clear them and they will go scot-free in spite of their sinfulness. Such are some of the various motives for work.

Work for work's sake. There are some who are really the salt of the earth in every country

and who work for work's sake, who do not care
for name, or fame, or even to go to heaven.
They work just because good will come of it.
There are others who do good to the poor and
help mankind from still higher motives, because
they believe in doing good and love good. The
motive for name and fame seldom brings imme-
diate results as a rule; they come to us when we
are old and have almost done with life. If a man
works without any selfish motive in view, does
he not gain anything? Yes, he gains the highest.
Unselfishness is more paying, only people have
not the patience to practise it. It is more paying
from the point of view of health also. Love,
truth, and unselfishness are not merely moral
figures of speech, but they form our highest
ideal, because in them lies such a manifestation
of power. In the first place, a man who can work
for five days or even for five minutes without
any selfish motive whatever, without thinking of
future, of heaven, of punishment, or anything of
the kind, has in him the capacity to become a
powerful moral giant. It is hard to do it, but in
the heart of our hearts we know its value, and
the good it brings. It is the greatest manifestation of power—this tremendous restraint; self-
restraint is a manifestation of greater power than
all outgoing action. A carriage with four horses
may rush down a hill unrestrained, or the coach-

man may curb the horses. Which is the greater manifestation of power, to let them go or to hold them? A cannon-ball flying through the air goes a long distance and falls. Another is cut short in its flight by striking against a wall, and the impact generates intense heat. All outgoing energy following a selfish motive is frittered away; it will not cause power to return to you; but if restrained, it will result in development of power. This self-control will tend to produce a mighty will, a character which makes a Christ or a Buddha. Foolish men do not know this secret; they nevertheless want to rule mankind. Even a fool may rule the whole world if he works and waits. Let him wait a few years, restrain that foolish idea of governing; and when that idea is wholly gone, he will be a power in the world. The majority of us cannot see beyond a few years, just as some animals cannot see beyond a few steps. Just a little narrow circle— that is our world. We have not the patience to look beyond, and thus become immoral and wicked. This is our weakness, our powerlessness.

Even the lowest forms of work are not to be despised. Let the man who knows no better, work for selfish ends, for name and fame; but everyone should always try to get towards higher and higher motives and to understand them. "To work we have the right, but not to the fruits thereof." Leave the fruits alone. Why care for results? If you wish to help a man, never think what that man's attitude should be towards you. If you want to do a great or a good work, do not trouble to think what the result will be.

There arises a difficult question in this ideal of work. Intense activity is necessary; we must always work. We cannot live a minute without work. What then becomes of rest? Here is one side of the life-struggle—work, in which we are whirled rapidly round. And here is the other, that of calm, retiring renunciation; everything is peaceful around, there is very little of noise and show, only nature with her animals and flowers and mountains. Neither of them is a perfect picture. A man used to solitude, if brought in contact with the surging whirlpool of the world, will be crushed by it; just as the fish that lives in the deep sea water, as soon as it is brought to the surface, breaks into pieces, deprived of the weight of water on it that had kept it together. Can a man who has been used to the turmoil and the rush of life live at ease if he comes to a quiet place? He suffers and perchance may lose his mind. The ideal man is he who in the midst of the greatest silence and solitude finds the intensest activity, and in the midst of the intensest activity finds the silence and solitude of the desert. He has learnt the secret of restraint, he has controlled himself. He goes through the streets of a big city with all its traffic, and his mind is as calm as if he were in a cave where not a sound could reach him; and he is intensely working all the time. That is the ideal of Karma-Yoga; and if you have attained to that, you have really learnt the secret of work.

But we have to begin from the beginning, to take up the works as they come to us and slowly make ourselves more unselfish every day. We must do the work and find out the motive power that prompts us; and, almost without exception, in the first years we shall find that our motives are always selfish; but gradually this selfishness will melt by persistence, till at last will come the time when we shall be able to do really unselfish work. We may all hope that some day or other, as we struggle through the paths of life, there will come a time when we shall become perfectly unselfish; and the moment we attain to that, all our powers will be concentrated, and the knowledge which is ours will be manifest.

EACH IS GREAT IN HIS OWN PLACE

ACCORDING to the Sânkhya philosophy, nature is composed of three forces called, in Sanskrit, Sattva, Rajas and Tamas. These as manifested in the physical world are what we may call equilibrium, activity, and inertness. Tamas is typified as darkness or inactivity; Rajas is activity, expressed as attraction or repulsion; and Sattva is the equilibrum of the two.

In every man there are these three forces. Sometimes Tamas prevails. We become lazy, we cannot move, we are inactive, bound down by certain ideas or by mere dullness. At other times activity prevails, and at still other times that calm balancing of both. Again, in different men, one of these forces is generally predominant. The characteristic of one man is inactivity, dullness, and laziness; that of another, activity, power, manifestation of energy; and in still another we find the sweetness, calmness, and gentleness which are due to the balancing of both action and inaction. So in all creation— in animals, plants, and men—we find the more or less typical manifestation of all these different forces.

Karma-Yoga has specially to deal with these three factors. By teaching what they are and how to employ them, it helps us to do our work better. Human society is a graded organisation. We all know about morality, and we all know about duty, but at the same time we find that in different countries the significance of morality varies greatly. What is regarded as moral in one country, may in another be considered perfectly immoral. For instance, in one country cousins may marry; in another, it is thought to be very immoral; in one, men may marry their sisters-in-law; in another, it is regarded as immoral; in one country people may marry only once; in another, many times; and so forth. Similarly, in all other departments of morality, we find the standard varies greatly; yet we have the idea that there must be a universal standard of morality.

So it is with duty. The idea of duty varies much among different nations. In one country, if a man does not do certain things, people will say he has acted wrongly; while if he does those very things in another country, people will say that he did not act rightly—and yet we know that there must be some universal idea of duty. In the same way, one class of society thinks that certain things are among its duty, while another class thinks quite the opposite and would be horrified if it had to do those things. Two ways are left open to us—the way of the ignorant who think that there is only one way to truth and that all the rest are wrong, and the way of the wise who admit that, according to our mental constitution or the different planes of existence in which we are, duty and morality may vary. The important thing is to know that there are gradations of duty and of morality— that the duty of one state of life, in one set of circumstances, will not and cannot be that of another.

To illustrate: All great teachers have taught, "Resist not evil", that non-resistance is the highest moral ideal. We all know that if a certain number of us attempted to put that maxim fully into practice, the whole social fabric would fall to pieces, the wicked would take possession of our properties and our lives, and would do whatever they liked with us. Even if for only one day such non-resistance were practised, it would lead to disaster. Yet, intuitively, in our heart of hearts we feel the truth of the teaching, "Resist not evil". This seems to us to be the highest ideal; yet to teach this doctrine only would be equivalent to condemning a vast portion of mankind. Not only so, it would be making men feel that they were always doing wrong, and cause in them scruples of conscience in all their actions; it would weaken them, and that constant self-disapproval would breed more vice than any other weakness would. To the man who has begun to hate himself the gate to degeneration has already opened; and the same is true of a nation.

Our first duty is not to hate ourselves; because to advance we must have faith in ourselves first and then in God. He who has no faith in himself can never have faith in God. Therefore the only alternative remaining to us is to recognise that duty and morality vary under different circumstances; not that the man who resists evil is doing what is always and in itself wrong, but that in the different circumstances in which he is placed it may become even his duty to resist evil.

In reading the Bhagavad-Gita, many of you in Western countries may have felt astonished at the second chapter, wherein Shri Krishna calls Arjuna a hypocrite and a coward because of his refusal to fight or offer resistance on account of his adversaries being his friends and relatives, making the plea that non-resistance was the highest ideal of love. This is a great lesson for us all to learn, that in all matters the two extremes are alike; the extreme positive and the extreme negative are always similar; when the vibrations of light are too slow we do not see them, nor do we see them when they are too rapid. So with sound; when very low in pitch we do not hear it, when very high we do not

hear it either. Of like nature is the difference
between resistance and non-resistance. One man
does not resist because he is weak, lazy, and
cannot, not because he will not; the other man
knows that he can strike an irresistible blow if
he likes; yet he not only does not strike, but
blesses his enemies. The one who from weakness
resists not commits a sin, and as such cannot
receive any benefit from the non-resistance;
while the other would commit a sin by offering
resistance. Buddha gave up his throne and renounced his position; that was true renunciation.
But there cannot be any question of renunciation
in the case of a beggar who has nothing to
renounce. So we must always be careful about
what we really mean when we speak of this
non-resistance and ideal love. We must first
take care to understand whether we have the
power of resistance or not. Then, having the
power, if we renounce it and do not resist, we
are doing a grand act of love; but if we cannot
resist, and yet, at the same time, try to deceive
ourselves into the belief that we are actuated
by motives of the highest love, we are doing
the exact opposite. Arjuna became a coward at
the sight of the mighty array against him; his
"love" made him forget his duty towards his
country and king. That is why Shri Krishna told
him that he was a hypocrite: Thou talkest like

a wise man, but thy actions betray thee to be a coward; therefore stand up and fight!

Such is the central idea of Karma-Yoga. The Karma-Yogi is the man who understands that the highest ideal is non-resistance, and who also knows that this non-resistance is the highest manifestation of power in actual possession, and also what is called the resisting of evil is but a step on the way towards the manifestation of this highest power, namely, non-resistance. Before reaching this highest ideal, man's duty is to resist evil; let him work, let him fight, let him strike straight from the shoulder. Then only, when he has gained the power to resist, will non-resistance be a virtue.

I once met a man in my country whom I had known before as a very stupid, dull person, who knew nothing and had not the desire to know anything, and was living the life of a brute. He asked me what he should do to know God, how he was to get free. "Can you tell a lie?" I asked him. "No," he replied. "Then you must learn to do so. It is better to tell a lie than to be a brute or a log of wood. You are inactive; you have not certainly reached the highest state, which is beyond all actions, calm and serene; you are too dull even to do something wicked." That was an extreme case, of course, and I was joking with him; but what I meant was that a man must be active in order to pass through activity to perfect calmness.

Inactivity should be avoided by all means. Activity always means resistance. Resist all evils, mental and physical; and when you have suc ceeded in resisting, then will calmness come. It is very easy to say, "Hate nobody, resist not evil", but we know what that kind of thing generally means in practice. When the eyes of society are turned towards us, we may make a show of non-resistance, but in our hearts it is canker all the time. We feel the utter want of the calm of non-resistance; we feel that it would be better for us to resist. If you desire wealth, and know at the same time that the whole world regards him who aims at wealth as a very wicked man, you, perhaps, will not dare to plunge into the struggle for wealth, yet your mind will be running day and night after money. This is hypocrisy and will serve no purpose. Plunge into the world, and then, after a time, when you have suffered and enjoyed all that is in it, will renunciation come; then will calmness come. So fulfil your desire for power and everything else, and after you have fulfilled the desire, will come the time when you will know that they are all very little things; but until you have fulfilled this desire, until you have passed through that activity, it is impossible for you to come to the state of calmness, serenity, and self-surrender. These ideas of serenity and renunciation have been preached for thousands of years; everybody has heard of them from childhood, and yet we see very few in the world who have really reached that stage. I do not know if I have seen twenty persons in my life who are really calm and non-resisting, and I have travelled over half the world.

Every man should take up his own ideal and endeavour to accomplish it; that is a surer way of progress than taking up other men's ideals which he can never hope to accomplish. For instance, we take a child and at once give him the task of walking twenty miles. Either the little one dies, or one in a thousand crawls the twenty miles to reach the end exhausted and half-dead. That is like what we generally try to do with the world. All the men and women in any society are not of the same mind, capacity, or of the same power to do things; they must have different ideals, and we have no right to sneer at any ideal. Let everyone do the best he can for realising his own ideal. Nor is it right that I should be judged by your standard or you by mine. The apple tree should not be judged by the standard of the oak, nor the oak by that of the apple. To judge the apple tree you must take the apple standard, and for the oak its own standard.

Unity in variety is the plan of creation. However men and women may vary individually, there is unity in the background. The different individual characters and classes of men and women are natural variations in creation. Hence we ought not to judge them by the same standard or put the same ideal before them. Such a course creates only an unnatural struggle, and the result is that man begins to hate himself and is hindered from becoming religious and good. Our duty is to encourage everyone in his struggle to live up to his own highest ideal, and strive at the same time to make the ideal as near as possible to the truth.

In the Hindu system of morality we find that this fact has been recognised from very ancient times and in their scriptures and books on ethics different rules are laid down for the different classes of men—the householder, the Sannyâsin (the man who has renounced the world), and the student.

The life of every individual, according to the Hindu scriptures, has its peculiar duties apart from what belongs in common to universal humanity. The Hindu begins life as a student; then he marries and becomes a householder; in old age he retires, and lastly he gives up the world and becomes a Sannyasin. To each of these stages of life certain duties are attached. No one of these stages is intrinsically superior to another. The life of the married man is quite as great as that of the celibate who has devoted himself to religious work. The scavenger in the street is quite as great and glorious as the king on his throne. Take him off his throne, make him do the work of the scavenger, and see how he fares. Take up the scavenger and see how he will rule. It is useless to say that the man who lives out of the world is a greater man than he who lives in the world; it is much more difficult to live in the world and worship God than to give it up and live a free and easy life. The four stages of life in India have in later times been reduced to two—that of the householder and of the monk. The householder marries and carries on his duties as a citizen, and the duty of the other is to devote his energies wholly to religion, to preach and to worship God. I shall read to you a few passages from the *Mahâ-Nirvâna-Tantra*, which treats of this subject, and you will see that it is a very difficult task for a man to be a householder, and perform all his duties perfectly.

The householder should be devoted to God; the knowledge of God should be his goal of life. Yet he must work constantly, perform all his duties; he must give up the fruits of his actions to God.

It is the most difficult thing in this world, to work and not care for the result, to help a man and never think that he ought to be grateful, to do some good work and at the same time never look to see whether it brings you name or fame, or nothing at all. Even the most arrant coward becomes brave when the world praises him. A fool can do heroic deeds when the approbation of society is upon him, but for a man to constantly do good without caring for the approbation of his fellowmen is indeed the highest sacrifice man can perform. The great duty of the householder is to earn a living, but he must take care that he does not do it by telling lies, or by cheating, or by robbing others; and he must remember that his life is for the service of God and the poor.

Knowing that mother and father are the visible representatives of God, the householder, always and by all means, must please them. If the mother is pleased, and the father, God is pleased with the man. That child is really a good child who never speaks harsh words to his parents.

Before parents one must not utter jokes, must not show restlessness, must not show anger or temper. Before mother or father, a child must bow down low, and stand up in their presence, and must not take a seat until they order him to sit.

If the householder has food and drink and clothes without first seeing that his mother and his father, his children, his wife, and the poor are supplied, he is committing a sin. The mother and the father are the causes of this body, so a man must undergo a thousand troubles in order to do good to them.

Even so is his duty to his wife; no man should scold his wife, and he must always maintain her as if she were his own mother. And even when he is in the greatest difficulties and troubles, he must not show anger to his wife.

He who thinks of another woman besides his wife, if he touches her even with his mind—that man goes to dark hell.

Before women he must not talk improper language, and never brag of his powers. He must not say, "I have done this, and I have done that."

The householder must always please his wife with money, clothes, love, faith, and words like nectar, and never do anything to disturb her. That man who has succeeded in getting the love of a chaste wife has succeeded in his religion and has all the virtues.

The following are duties towards children:

A son should be lovingly reared up to his

fourth year; he should be educated till he is sixteen. When he is twenty years of age he should be employed in some work; he should then be treated affectionately by his father as his equal. Exactly in the same manner the daughter should be brought up, and should be educated with the greatest care. And when she marries, the father ought to give her jewels and wealth.

Then the duty of the man is towards his brothers and sisters, and towards the children of his brothers and sisters, if they are poor, and towards his other relatives, his friends, and his servants. Then his duties are towards the people of the same village, and the poor, and anyone that comes to him for help. Having sufficient means, if the householder does not take care to give to his relatives and to the poor, know him to be only a brute; he is not a human being.

Excessive attachment to food, clothes, and the tending of the body, and dressing of the hair should be avoided. The householder must be pure in heart and clean in body, always active and always ready for work.

To his enemies the householder must be a hero. Them he must resist. That is the duty of the householder. He must not sit down in a corner and weep, and talk nonsense about non-resistance. If he does not show himself a hero to his enemies he has not done his duty. And to his friends and relatives he must be as gentle as a lamb.

It is the duty of the householder not to pay reverence to the wicked; because, if he reverences the wicked people of the world, he patronises wickedness; and it will be a great mistake if he disregards those who are worthy of respect, the good people. He must not be gushing in his friendship; he must not go out of the way making friends everywhere; he must watch the actions of the men he wants to make friends with, and their dealings with other men, reason upon them, and then make friends.

These three things he must not talk of. He must not talk in public of his own fame; he must not preach his own name or his own powers; he must not talk of his wealth, or of anything that has been told to him privately.

A man must not say he is poor, or that he is wealthy—he must not brag of his wealth. Let him keep his own counsel; this is his religious duty. This is not mere worldly wisdom; if a man does not do so, he may be held to be immoral.

The householder is the basis, the prop of the whole society; he is the principal earner. The poor, the weak, the children, and the women who do not work—all live upon the householder; so there must be certain duties that he has to perform, and these duties must make him feel strong to perform them, and not make him think that he is doing things beneath his ideal. Therefore, if he has done something weak or has made some mistake, he must not say so in public; and if he is engaged in some enterprise and knows he is sure to fail in it, he must not speak of it. Such self-exposure is not only uncalled for, but also unnerves the man and makes him unfit for the performance of his legitimate duties in life. At the same time, he must struggle hard to acquire these things—first, knowledge, and secondly, wealth. It is his duty; and if he does not do his duty, he is nobody. A householder who does not struggle to get wealth is immoral. If he is lazy and content to lead an idle life, he is immoral, because upon him depend hundreds. If he gets riches, hundreds of others will be thereby supported.

If there were not in this city hundreds who had striven to become rich, and who had acquired wealth, where would all this civilisation, and these alms-houses and great houses be?

Going after wealth in such a case is not bad, because that wealth is for distribution. The householder is the centre of life and society. It is a worship for him to acquire and spend wealth nobly, for the householder who struggles

to become rich by *good* means and for *good*
purposes is doing practically the same thing for
the attainment of salvation as the anchorite does
in his cell when he is praying, for in them we
see only the different aspects of the same virtue
of self-surrender and self-sacrifice prompted by
the feeling of devotion to God and to all that is
His.

He must struggle to acquire a good name by
all means. He must not gamble, he must not
move in the company of the wicked, he must
not tell lies, and must not be the cause of
trouble to others.

Often people enter into things they have not
the means to accomplish, with the result that
they cheat others to attain their own ends. Then
there is in all things the time factor to be taken
into consideration; what at one time might be a
failure, would perhaps at another time be a very
great success.

The householder must speak the truth and
speak gently, using words which people like,
which will do good to others; nor should he
talk of the business of other men.

The householder by digging tanks, by planting
trees on the roadsides, by establishing rest-
houses for men and animals, by making roads
and building bridges, goes towards the same
goal as the greatest Yogi.

This is one part of the doctrine of Karma-Yoga
—activity, the duty of the householder. There is
a passage later on, where it says that "if the
householder dies in battle fighting for his country or his religion, he comes to the same goal
as the Yogi by meditation", showing thereby
that what is duty for one is not duty for another.
At the same time, it does not say that this duty
is lowering and the other elevating. Each duty
has its own place, and according to the circumstances in which we are placed, must we
perform our duties.

One idea comes out of all this, the condem-
nation of all weakness. This is a particular idea
in all our teachings which I like, either in
philosophy, or in religion, or in work. If you
read the Vedas, you will find this word always
repeated—"fearlessness"—fear nothing. Fear is
a sign of weakness. A man must go about his
duties without taking notice of the sneers and
the ridicule of the world.

If a man retires from the world to worship
God, he must not think that those who live in
the world and work for the good of the world
are not worshipping God; neither must those
who live in the world for wife and children
think that those who give up the world are low
vagabonds. Each is great in his own place. This
thought I will illustrate by a story.

A certain king used to inquire of all the Sannyasins that came to his country, "Which is the greater man—he who gives up the world and becomes a Sannyasin, or he who lives in the world and performs his duties as a householder?" Many wise men sought to solve the problem. Some asserted that the Sannyasin was the greater, upon which the king demanded that they should prove their assertion. When they could not, he ordered them to marry and become householders. Then others came and said, "The householder who performs his duties is the greater man." Of them, too, the king demanded proofs. When they could not give them, he made them also settle down as householders.

At last there came a young Sannyasin, and the king similarly inquired of him also. He answered, "Each, O king, is equally great in his place." "Prove this to me", asked the king. "I will prove it to you", said the Sannyasin, "but you must first come and live as I do for a few days, that I may be able to prove to you what I say." The king consented and followed the Sannyasin out of his own territory and passed through many other countries until they came to a great kingdom. In the capital of that kingdom a great ceremony was going on. The king and the Sannyasin heard the noise of drums and music, and heard also the criers; the people were assembled in the streets in gala dress, and a great proclamation was being made. The king and the Sannyasin stood there to see what was going on. The crier was proclaiming loudly that the princess, daughter of the king of that country, was about to choose a husband from among those assembled before her.

It was an old custom in India for princesses to choose husbands in this way. Each princess had certain ideas of the sort of man she wanted for a husband; some would have the handsomest man; others would have only the most learned; others again the richest, and so on. All the princes of the neighbourhood put on their bravest attire and presented themselves before her. Sometimes they too had their own criers to enumerate their advantages and the reasons why they hoped the princess would choose them. The princess was taken round on a throne in the most splendid array and looked at and heard about them. If she was not pleased with what she saw and heard, she said to her bearers, "Move on", and no more notice was taken of the rejected suitors. If, however, the princess was pleased with any one of them, she threw a garland of flowers over him, and he became her husband.

The princess of the country to which our king and the Sannyasin had come was having one of these interesting ceremonies. She was the most beautiful princess in the world, and the husband of the princess would be ruler of the kingdom after her father's death. The idea of this princess was to marry the handsomest man, but she could not find the right one to please her. Several times these meetings had taken place, but the princess could not select a husband. This meeting was the most splendid of all; more people than ever had come to it. The princess came in on a throne, and the bearers carried her from place to place. She did not seem to care for anyone, and everyone became disappointed that this meeting also was going to be a failure. Just then came a young man, a Sannyasin, handsome as if the sun had come down to the earth, and stood in one corner of the assembly watching what was going on. The throne with the princess came near him, and as soon as she saw the beautiful Sannyasin, she stopped and threw the garland over him. The young Sannyasin seized the garland and threw it off, exclaiming, "What nonsense is this? I am a Sannyasin. What is marriage to me?" The king of that country thought that perhaps this man was poor and so dared not marry the princess, and said to him, "With my daughter goes half my kingdom now, and the whole kingdom after my death!" and put the garland again on the Sannyasin. The young man threw it off once more, saying, "Nonsense! I do not want to marry", and walked quickly away from the assembly.

Now the princess had fallen so much in love with this young man that she said, "I must marry this man or I shall die". And she went after him to bring him back. Then our other Sannyasin, who had brought the king there said to him, "King, let us follow this pair". So they walked after them but at a good distance behind. The young Sannyasin who had refused to marry the princess walked out into the country for several miles. When he came to a forest and entered into it, the princess followed him, and the other two followed them. Now this young Sannyasin was well acquainted with that forest and knew all the intricate paths in it. He suddenly passed into one of these and disappeared, and the princess could not discover him. After trying for a long time to find him, she sat down under a tree and began to weep, for she did not know the way out. Then our king and the other Sannyasin came up to her and said, "Do not weep; we will show you the way out of this forest, but it is too dark for us to find it now. Here is a big tree; let us rest under it, and in the morning we will go early and show you the road."

Now a little bird and his wife and their three

little ones lived on that tree in a nest. This little bird looked down and saw the three people under the tree and said to his wife, "My dear, what shall we do? Here are some guests in the house, and it is winter, and we have no fire." So he flew away and got a bit of burning firewood in his beak and dropped it before the guests, to which they added fuel and made a blazing fire. But the little bird was not satisfied. He said again to his wife, "My dear, what shall we do? There is nothing to give these people to eat, and they are hungry. We are householders; it is our duty to feed anyone who comes to the house. I must do what I can, I will give them my body." So he plunged into the midst of the fire and perished. The guests saw him falling and tried to save him, but he was too quick for them.

The little bird's wife saw what her husband did, and she said, "Here are three persons and only one little bird for them to eat. It is not enough; it is my duty as a wife not to let my husband's effort go in vain; let them have my body also." Then she fell into the fire and was burned to death.

Then the three baby-birds, when they saw what was done and that there was still not enough food for the three guests, said, "Our parents have done what they could and still it is not enough. It is our duty to carry on the

work of our parents; let our bodies go too."
And they all dashed down into the fire also.

Amazed at what they saw, the three people
could not of course eat these birds. They passed
the night without food, and in the morning the
king and the Sannyasin showed the princess the
way, and she went back to her father.

Then the Sannyasin said to the king, "King,
you have seen that each is great in his own
place. If you want to live in the world, live like
those birds, ready at any moment to sacrifice
yourself for others. If you want to renounce the
world, be like that young man to whom the
most beautiful woman and a kingdom were as
nothing. If you want to be householder, hold
your life a sacrifice for the welfare of others;
and if you choose the life of renunciation, do
not even look at beauty, and money, and power.
Each is great in his own place, but the duty of
the one is not the duty of the other."

THE SECRET OF WORK

HELPING others physically, by removing their physical needs, is indeed great; but the help is greater according as the need is greater and according as the help is far-reaching. If a man's wants can be removed for an hour, it is helping him indeed; if his wants can be removed for a year, it will be more help to him; but if his wants can be removed for ever, it is surely the greatest help that can be given him. Spiritual knowledge is the only thing that can destroy our miseries for ever; any other knowledge satisfies wants only for a time. It is only with the knowledge of the spirit that the faculty of want is annihilated for ever; so helping man spiritually is the highest help that can be given him. He who gives man spiritual knowledge is the greatest benefactor of mankind, and as such we always find that those were the most powerful of men who helped man in his spiritual needs, because spirituality is the true basis of all our activities in life. A spiritually strong and sound man will be strong in every other respect, if he so wishes; until there is spiritual strength in man even physical needs cannot be well satisfied. Next to spiritual comes intellectual help; the gift of knowledge is a far higher gift than that of food and clothes; it is even higher than giving life to a man, because the real life of man consists of knowledge. Ignorance is death, knowledge is life. Life is of very little value, if it is a life in the dark, groping through ignorance and misery. Next in order comes, of course, helping a man physically. Therefore, in considering the question of helping others, we must always strive not to commit the mistake of thinking that physical help is the only help that can be given. It is not only the last but the least, because it cannot bring about permanent satisfaction. The misery that I feel when I am hungry is satisfied by eating, but hunger returns; my misery can cease only when I am satisfied beyond all want. Then hunger will not make me miserable; no distress, no sorrow will be able to move me. So that help which tends to make us strong spiritually is the highest, next to it comes intellectual help, and after that physical help.

The miseries of the world cannot be cured by physical help only. Until man's nature changes, these physical needs will always arise, and miseries will always be felt, and no amount of physical help will cure them completely. The only solution of this problem is to make mankind pure. Ignorance is the mother of all the evil and all the misery we see. Let men have light, let them be pure and spiritually strong and educated, then alone will misery cease in the world, not before. We may convert every house in the country into a charity asylum; we may fill the land with hospitals, but the misery of man will still continue to exist until man's character changes.

We read in the Bhagavad-Gita again and again that we must all work incessantly. All work is by nature composed of good and evil. We cannot do any work which will not do some good somewhere; there cannot be any work which will not cause some harm somewhere. Every work must necessarily be a mixture of good and evil; yet we are commanded to work incessantly. Good and evil will both have their results, will produce their Karma. Good action will entail upon us good effect; bad action, bad. But good and bad are both bondages of the soul. The solution reached in the Gita in regard to this bondage-producing nature of work is, that if we do not attach ourselves to the work we do, it will not have any binding effect on our soul. We shall try to understand what is meant by this "non-attachment" to work.

This is the one central idea in the Gita: Work incessantly, but be not attached to it. "Samskâra" can be translated very nearly by inherent tendency. Using the simile of a lake for the mind, every ripple, every wave that rises in the mind, when it subsides, does not die out entirely, but leaves a mark and a future possibility of that wave coming out again. This mark, with the possibility of the wave reappearing, is what is called Samskara. Every work that we do, every movement of the body, every thought that we think, leaves such an impression on the mind-stuff, and even when such impressions are not obvious on the surface, they are sufficiently strong to work beneath the surface subconsciously. What we are every moment is determined by the sum total of these impressions on the mind. What I am just at this moment is the effect of the sum total of all the impressions of my past life. This is really what is meant by character; each man's character is determined by the sum total of these impressions. If good impressions prevail, the character becomes good; if bad, it becomes bad. If a man continuously hears bad words, thinks bad thoughts, does bad actions, his mind will be full of bad impressions; and they will influence his thought and work without his being conscious of the fact. In fact, these bad impressions are always working, and their resultant must be evil; and that man will be a bad man, he cannot help it. The sum total of these impressions in him will create the strong motive power for doing bad actions. He will be like a machine in the hands of his impressions, and they will force him to do evil. Similarly, if a man thinks good thoughts and does good works, the sum total of these impressions will be good; and they, in a similar manner, will force him to do good even in spite of himself. When a man has done so much good work and thought so many good thoughts that there is an irresistible tendency in him to do good, in spite of himself and even if he wishes to do evil, his mind, as the sum total of his tendencies, will not allow him to do so; the tendencies will turn him back; he is completely under the influence of the good tendencies. When such is the case, a man's good character is said to be established.

As the tortoise tucks its feet and head inside the shell, and you may kill it and break it in pieces, and yet it will not come out, even so the character of that man who has control over his motives and organs is unchangeably established. He controls his own inner forces, and nothing can draw them out against his will. By this continuous reflex of good thoughts, good impressions moving over the surface of the mind, the tendency for doing good becomes strong, and as the result we feel able to control the Indriyas (the sense-organs, the nerve-centres). Thus alone will character be established, then alone a man gets to truth. Such a man is safe for ever; he cannot do any evil. You may place him in any company, there will be no danger for him. There is a still higher state than having this good tendency, and that is the desire for liberation. You must remember that freedom of the soul is the goal of all Yogas, and each one equally leads to the same result. By work alone men may get to where Buddha got largely by meditation or Christ by prayer. Buddha was a working Jnani; Christ was a Bhakta. But the same goal was reached by both of them. The difficulty is here. Liberation means entire freedom—freedom from the bondage of good, as well as from the bondage of evil. A golden chain is as much a chain as an iron one. There is a thorn in my finger, and I use another to take the first one out; and when I have taken it out, I throw both of them aside; I have no necessity for keeping the second thorn, because both are thorns after all. So the bad tendencies are to be counteracted by the good ones, and the bad impressions on the mind should be removed by the fresh waves of good ones, until all that is evil almost disappears, or is subdued and held in control in a corner of the mind; but after that, the good tendencies have also to be conquered. Thus the "attached" becomes the "unattached". Work, but let not the action or the thought produce a deep impression on the mind; let the ripples come and go; let huge actions proceed from the muscles and the brain, but let them not make any deep impression on the soul.

How can this be done? We see that the impression of any action to which we attach ourselves, remains. I may meet hundreds of persons during the day, and among them meet also one whom I love; and when I retire at night, I may try to think of all the faces I saw, but only that face comes before the mind—the face which I met perhaps only for one minute, and which I loved; all the others have vanished. My attachment to this particular person caused a deeper impression on my mind than all the other faces. Physiologically, the impressions have all been the same; every one of the faces that I saw pictured itself on the retina, and the brain took the pictures in; and yet there was no similarity of effect upon the mind. Most of the faces, perhaps, were entirely new faces, about which I had never thought before; but that one face of which I got only a glimpse, found associations inside. Perhaps I had pictured him in my mind for years, knew hundreds of things about him, and this one new vision of him awakened hundreds of sleeping memories in my mind; and this one impression having been repeated perhaps a hundred times more than those of the different faces together, will produce a great effect on the mind.

Therefore, be "unattached", let things work; let brain centres work; work incessantly, but let not a ripple conquer the mind. Work as if you were a stranger in this land, a sojourner; work incessantly, but do not bind yourselves; bondage is terrible. This world is not our habitation, it is only one of the many stages through which we are passing. Remember that great saying of the Sânkhya, "The whole of nature is for the soul, not the soul for nature." The very reason of nature's existence is for the education of the soul; it has no other meaning; it is there because the soul must have knowledge and through knowledge free itself. If we remember this always, we shall never be attached to nature; we shall know that nature is a book in which we are to read, and that when we have gained the required knowledge, the book is of no more value to us. Instead of that, however, we are identifying ourselves with nature; we are thinking that the soul is for nature, that the spirit is for the flesh, and, as the common saying has it, we think that man "lives to eat" and not "eats to live". We are continually making this mistake; we are regarding nature as ourselves and are becoming attached to it; and as soon as this attachment comes, there is the deep impression on the soul, which binds us down and makes us work not from freedom but like slaves.

The whole gist of this teaching is that you should work like a *master* and not as a *slave*; work incessantly, but do not do slave's work. Do you not see how everybody works? Nobody can be altogether at rest; ninety-nine per cent of mankind work like slaves, and the result is misery; it is all selfish work. Work through freedom! Work through love! The word "love" is very difficult to understand; love never comes until there is freedom. There is no true love possible in the slave. If you buy a slave and tie him down in chains and make him work for you, he will work like a drudge, but there will be no love in him. So when we ourselves work for the things of the world as slaves, there can be no love in us, and our work is not true work. This is true of work done for relatives and friends, and is true of work done for our own selves. Selfish work is slave's work; and here is a test. Every act of love brings happiness; there is no act of love which does not bring peace and blessedness as its reaction. Real existence, real knowledge, and real love are eternally connected with one another, the three in one: where one of them is, the others also must be; they are the three aspects of the One without a second—the Existence-Knowledge-Bliss. When that existence becomes relative, we see it as the world; that knowledge becomes in its turn modified into the knowledge of the things of the world; and that bliss forms the foundation of all true love known to the heart of man. Therefore true love can never react so as to cause pain either to the lover or to the beloved. Suppose a man loves a woman; he wishes to have her all to himself and feels extremely jealous about her every movement; he wants her to sit near him, to stand near him, and to eat and move at his bidding. He is a slave to her and wishes to have her as his slave. That is not love; it is a kind of morbid affection of the slave, insinuating itself as love. It cannot be love, because it is painful; if she does not do what he wants, it brings him pain. With love there is no painful reaction; love only brings a reaction of bliss; if it does not, it is not love; it is mistaking something else for love. When you have succeeded in loving your husband, your wife, your children, the whole world, the universe in such a manner that there is no reaction of pain or jealousy, no selfish feeling, then you are in a fit state to be unattached.

Krishna says, "Look at Me, Arjuna! If I stop from work for one moment, the whole universe will die. I have nothing to gain from work; I am the one Lord, but why do I work? Because I love the world." God is unattached because He loves; that real love makes us unattached. Wherever there is attachment, the clinging to the things of the world, you must know that it is all physical attraction between sets of particles of matter; something that attracts two bodies nearer and nearer all the time and, if they cannot get near enough, produces pain; but where there is *real* love, it does not rest on physical attachment at all. Such lovers may be a thousand miles away from one another, but their love will be all the same; it does not die, and will never produce any painful reaction.

To attain this non-attachment is almost a life-work. But as soon as we have reached this point, we have attained the goal of love and become free; the bondage of nature falls from us, and we see nature as she is; she forges no more chains for us; we stand entirely free and take not the results of work into consideration; who then cares for what the results may be?

Do you ask anything from your children in return for what you have given them? It is your duty to work for them, and there the matter ends. In whatever you do for a particular person, a city, or a state, assume the same attitude towards it as you have towards your children— expect nothing in return. If you can invariably take the position of a giver, in which everything given by you is a free offering to the world without any thought of return, then will your work bring you no attachment. Attachment comes only where we expect a return.

If working like slaves results in selfishness and attachment, working as masters of our own mind gives rise to the bliss of non-attachment. We often talk of right and justice, but we find that in the world right and justice are mere baby's talk. There are two things which guide the conduct of men: might and mercy. The exercise of might is invariably the exercise of selfishness. All men and women try to make the most of whatever power or advantage they have. Mercy is heaven itself; to be good we have all to be merciful. Even justice and right should stand on mercy. All thought of obtaining return for the work we do hinders our spiritual progress; nay, in the end it brings misery. There is another way in which this idea of mercy and selfless charity can be put into practice; that is, by looking upon work as "worship" in case we believe in a Personal God. Here we give up all the fruits of our work unto the Lord, and worshipping Him thus, we have no right to expect anything from mankind for the work we do. The Lord Himself works incessantly and is ever without attachment. Just as water cannot wet the lotus leaf, so work cannot bind the unselfish man by giving rise to attachment to results. The selfless and unattached man may live in the very heart of a crowded and sinful city; he will not be touched by sin.

This idea of complete self-sacrifice is illustrated in the following story: After the battle of Kurukshetra the five Pândava brothers performed a great sacrifice and made very large gifts to the poor. All people expressed amazement at the greatness and richness of the sacrifice, and said that such a sacrifice the world had never seen before. But, after the ceremony, there came a little mongoose; half his body was golden, and the other half was brown; and he began to roll on the floor of the sacrificial hall. He said to those around, "You are all liars; this is no sacrifice." "What!" they exclaimed, "you say this is no sacrifice; do you not know how money and jewels were poured out to the poor and everyone became rich and happy? This was the most wonderful sacrifice any man ever performed." But the mongoose said, "There was once a little village, and in it there dwelt a poor Brahmin with his wife, his son, and his son's wife. They were very poor and lived on small gifts made to them for preaching and teaching. There came in that land a three years' famine, and the poor Brahmin suffered more than ever. At last when the family had starved for days, the father brought home one morning a little barley flour, which he had been fortunate enough to

obtain, and he divided it into four parts, one for
each member of the family. They prepared it for
their meal, and just as they were about to eat
there was a knock at the door. The father
opened it, and there stood a guest. Now in India
a guest is a sacred person; he is as a god for the
time being, and must be treated as such. So the
poor Brahmin said, 'Come in, sir, you are wel-
come.' He set before the guest his own portion
of the food, which the guest quickly ate and
said, 'Oh, sir, you have killed me; I have been
starving for ten days, and this little bit has but
increased my hunger.' Then the wife said to her
husband, 'Give him my share'; but the husband
said, 'Not so.' The wife however insisted, saying, 'Here is a poor man, and it is our duty as
householders to see that he is fed, and it is my
duty as a wife to give him my portion, seeing
that you have no more to offer him.' Then she
gave her share to the guest, which he ate, and
said he was still burning with hunger. So the
son said, 'Take my portion also; it is the duty
of a son to help his father to fulfil his obliga-
tions.' The guest ate that, but remained still
unsatisfied; so the son's wife gave him her portion also. That was sufficient, and the guest
departed, blessing them. That night those four
people died of starvation. A few granules of that
flour had fallen on the floor, and when I rolled

my body on them, half of it became golden, as
you see. Since then I have been travelling all
over the world, hoping to find another sacrifice
like that, but nowhere have I found one; nowhere else has the other half of my body been
turned into gold. That is why I say this is no
sacrifice."

This idea of charity is going out of India;
great men are becoming fewer and fewer. When
I was first learning English, I read an English
story book in which there was a story about a
dutiful boy who had gone out to work and had
given some of his money to his old mother; and
this was praised in three or four pages. What
was that? No Hindu boy can ever understand
the moral of that story. Now I understand it
when I hear the Western idea—every man for
himself. And some men take everything for
themselves, and fathers and mothers and wives
and children go to the wall. That should never
and nowhere be the ideal of the householder.

Now you see what Karma-Yoga means; even
at the point of death to help anyone, without
asking questions. Be cheated millions of times
and never ask a question, and never think of
what you are doing. Never vaunt of your gifts
to the poor or expect their gratitude, but rather
be grateful to them for giving you the occasion
of practising charity to them. Thus it is plain

that to be an ideal householder is a much more difficult task than to be an ideal Sannyasin; the true life of work is indeed as hard as, if not harder than, the equally true life of renunciation.

WHAT IS DUTY?

IT is necessary in the study of Karma-Yoga to know what duty is. If I have to do something I must first know that it is my duty, and then I can do it. The idea of duty, again, is different in different nations. The Mohammedan says what is written in his book, the Koran, is his duty; the Hindu says what is in the Vedas is his duty; and the Christian says what is in the Bible is his duty. We find that there are varied ideas of duty, differing according to different states in life, different historical periods and different nations. The term "duty" like every other universal abstract term, is impossible clearly to define; we can only get an idea of it by knowing its practical operations and results. When certain things occur before us we have all a natural or trained impulse to act in a certain manner towards them; when this impulse comes, the mind begins to think about the situation. Sometimes it thinks that it is good to act in a particular manner under the given conditions, at other times it thinks that it is wrong to act in the same manner even in the very same circumstances. The ordinary idea of duty everywhere is that every good man follows the dictates of his conscience. But what is it that

makes an act a duty? If a Christian finds a piece
of beef before him and does not eat it to save
his own life or will not give it to save the life of
another man, he is sure to feel that he has not
done his duty. But if a Hindu dares to eat that
piece of beef or to give it to another Hindu, he
is equally sure to feel that he too has not done
his duty; the Hindu's training and education
make him feel that way. In the last century there
were notorious bands of robbers in India called
thugs; they thought it their duty to kill any man
they could and take away his money, the larger
the number of men they killed, the better they
thought they were. Ordinarily if a man goes out
into the street and shoots down another man, he
is apt to feel sorry for it, thinking that he has
done wrong. But if the very same man, as a
soldier in his regiment, kills not one but twenty,
he is certain to feel glad and think that he has
done his duty remarkably well. Therefore we see
that it is not the thing done that defines a duty.
To give an objective definition of duty is thus
entirely impossible. Yet there is duty from the
subjective side. Any action that makes us go
Godward is a good action, and is our duty; any
action that makes us go downward is evil and is
not our duty. From the subjective standpoint we
may see that certain acts have a tendency to
exalt and ennoble us, while certain other acts

have a tendency to degrade and to brutalise us. But it is not possible to make out with certainty which acts have which kind of tendency in relation to all persons of all sorts and conditions. There is, however, only one idea of duty which has been universally accepted by all mankind of all ages and sects and countries, and that has been summed up in a Sanskrit aphorism thus: "Do not injure any being; not injuring any being is virtue, injuring any being is sin."

The Bhagavad-Gita frequently alludes to duties dependent upon birth and position in life. Birth and position in life and in society largely determine the mental and moral attitude of individuals towards the various activities of life. It is therefore our duty to do that work which will exalt and ennoble us in accordance with the ideals and activities of the society in which we are born. But it must be particularly remembered that the same ideals and activities do not prevail in all societies and countries; our ignorance of this is the main cause of much of the hatred of one nation towards another. An American thinks that whatever an American does in accordance with the custom of his country is the best thing to do, and that whoever does not follow his custom must be a very wicked man. A Hindu thinks that his customs are the only right ones and are the best in the world, and that whosoever does not obey them must be the most wicked man living. This is quite a natural mistake which all of us are apt to make. But it is very harmful; it is the cause of half the uncharitableness found in the world. When I came to this country and was going through the Chicago Fair, a man from behind pulled at my turban. I looked back and saw that he was a very gentlemanly-looking man, neatly dressed. I spoke to him, and when he found that I knew English, he became very much abashed. On another occasion in the same Fair another man gave me a push. When I asked him the reason, he also was ashamed and stammered out an apology saying, "Why do you dress that way!" The sympathies of these men were limited within the range of their own language and their own fashion of dress. Much of the oppression of powerful nations on weaker ones is caused by this prejudice. It dries up their fellow-feeling for fellow-men. That very man who asked me why I did not dress as he did and wanted to ill-treat me because of my dress, may have been a very good man, a good father, and a good citizen; but the kindness of his nature died out as soon as he saw a man in a different dress. Strangers are exploited in all countries, because they do not know how to defend themselves; thus they carry home false impressions of the peoples they have seen. Sailors, soldiers, and traders behave in foreign lands in very queer ways, although they would not dream of doing so in their own country; perhaps this is why the Chinese call Europeans and Americans "foreign devils". They could not have done this if they had met the good, the kindly sides of Western life.

Therefore the one point we ought to remember is that we should always try to see the duty of others through their own eyes and never judge the customs of other peoples by our own standard. I am not the standard of the universe. I have to accommodate myself to the world, and not the world to me. So we see that environments change the nature of our duties, and doing the duty which is ours at any particular time is the best thing we can do in this world. Let us do that duty which is ours by birth; and when we have done that, let us do the duty which is ours by our position in life and in society. There is, however, one great danger in human nature, viz that man never examines himself. He thinks he is quite as fit to be on the throne as the king. Even if he is, he must first show that he has done the duty of his own position; and then higher duties will come to him. When we begin to work earnestly in the world, nature gives us blows right and left and soon enables us to find

out our position. No man can long occupy satis-
factorily a position for which he is not fit. There
is no use in grumbling against nature's adjust-
ment. He who does the lower work is not therefore a lower man. No man is to be judged by
the mere nature of his duties, but all should be
judged by the manner and the spirit in which
they perform them.

Later on we shall find that even this idea of
duty undergoes change, and that the greatest
work is done only when there is no selfish motive to prompt it. Yet it is work through the sense
of duty that leads us to work without any idea
of duty; when work will become worship—nay,
something higher—then will work be done for
its own sake. We shall find that the philosophy
of duty, whether it be in the form of ethics or
of love, is the same as in every other Yoga—the
object being the attenuating of the lower self so
that the real higher Self may shine forth, the
lessening of the frittering away of energies on
the lower plane of existence so that the soul
may manifest itself on the higher ones. This is
accomplished by the continuous denial of low
desires, which duty rigorously requires. The
whole organisation of society has thus been
developed consciously or unconsciously in the
realms of action and experience where, by limit-

ing selfishness, we open the way to an unlimited expansion of the real nature of man.

Duty is seldom sweet. It is only when love greases its wheels that it runs smoothly; it is a continuous friction otherwise. How else could parents do their duties to their children, husbands to their wives and vice versa? Do we not meet with cases of friction every day in our lives? Duty is sweet only through love, and love shines in freedom alone. Yet is it freedom to be a slave to the senses, to anger, to jealousies, and a hundred other petty things that must occur every day in human life? In all these little roughnesses that we meet with in life, the highest expression of freedom is to forbear. Women, slaves to their own irritable, jealous tempers, are apt to blame their husbands and assert their own "freedom", as they think, not knowing that thereby they only prove that they are slaves. So it is with husbands who eternally find fault with their wives.

Chastity is the first virtue in man or woman, and the man who, however he may have strayed away, cannot be brought to the right path by a gentle and loving and chaste wife, is indeed very rare. The world is not yet as bad as that. We hear much about brutal husbands all over the world and about the impurity of men, but is it not true that there are quite as many brutal and impure women as men? If all women were as good and pure as their own constant assertions would lead one to believe, I am perfectly satisfied that there would not be one impure man in the world. What brutality is there which purity and chastity cannot conquer? A good, chaste wife, who thinks of every other man except her own husband as her child and has the attitude of a mother towards all men, will grow so great in the power of her purity that there cannot be a single man, however brutal, who will not breathe an atmosphere of holiness in her presence. Similarly every husband, must look upon all women, except his own wife, in the light of his own mother or daughter or sister. That man, again, who wants to be a teacher of religion must look upon every woman as his mother and always behave towards her as such.

The position of the mother is the highest in the world, as it is the one place in which to learn and exercise the greatest unselfishness. The love of God is the only love that is higher than a mother's love; all others are lower. It is the duty of the mother to think of her children first and then of herself. But, instead of that, if the parents are always thinking of themselves first, the result is that the relation between parents and children becomes the same as that between birds and their offspring which, as soon

as they are fledged, do not recognise any parents.
Blessed indeed is the man who is able to look
upon woman as the representative of the mother-
hood of God. Blessed indeed is the woman to
whom man represents the fatherhood of God.
Blessed are the children who look upon their
parents as Divinity manifested on earth.

The only way to rise is by doing the duty next
to us, and thus we go on gathering strength
until we reach the highest state. A young Sannyasin went to a forest; there he meditated,
worshipped, and practised Yoga for a long time.
After years of hard work and practice, he was
one day sitting under a tree, when some dry
leaves fell upon his head. He looked up and saw
a crow and a crane fighting on the top of the
tree, which made him very angry. He said,
"What! Dare you throw these dry leaves upon
my head!" As with these words he angrily
glanced at them, a flash of fire went out of his
head—such was the Yogi's power—and burnt
the birds to ashes. He was very glad, almost
overjoyed at this development of power—he
could burn the crow and the crane by a
look. After a time he had to go to the town to
beg his bread. He went, stood at a door, and
said, "Mother, give me food." A voice came from
inside the house: "Wait a little, my son." The
young man thought: "You wretched woman,

how dare you make me wait! You do not know
my power yet." While he was thinking thus the
voice came again: "Boy, don't be thinking too
much of yourself. Here is neither crow nor
crane." He was astonished, still he had to wait.
At last woman came, and he fell at her feet
and said, "Mother, how did you know that?" She
said, "My boy, I do not know your Yoga or your
practices. I am a common everyday woman. I
made you wait because my husband was ill, and I
was nursing him. All my life I have struggled to
do my duty. When I was unmarried, I did my
duty to my parents; now that I am married, I
do my duty to my husband; that is all the Yoga
I practise. But by doing my duty I have become
illumined; thus I could read your thoughts and
know what you had done in the forest. If you
want to know something higher than this, go to
the market of such and such a town where you
will find a Vyâdha[1] who will tell you something
that you will be very glad to learn." The Sannyasin thought: "Why should I go to that town
and to a Vyadha!" But after what he had seen,
his mind opened a little, so he went. When he
came near the town, he found that market and
there saw at a distance a big fat Vyadha cutting
meat with big knives, talking and bargaining

[1] The lowest class of people in India, who used to
live as hunters and butchers.

KY-5

with different people. The young man said,
"Lord help me! Is this the man from whom I
am going to learn? He is the incarnation of a
demon, if he is anything." In the meantime this
man looked up and said, "O Swami, did that
lady send you here? Take a seat until I have
done my business." The Sannyasin thought,
"What comes to me here?" He took his seat; the
man went on with his work, and after he had
finished, he took his money and said to the Sannyasin, "Come, sir, come to my home." On reaching home the Vyadha gave him a seat, saying
"Wait here", and went into the house. He then
washed his old father and mother, fed them,
and did all he could to please them, after which
he came to the Sannyasin and said, "Now, sir,
you have come here to see me; what can I do
for you?" The Sannyasin asked him a few questions about soul and about God, and the Vyadha
gave him a lecture which forms a part of the
Mahâbhârata, called the Vyâdha-Gita. It con-
tains one of the highest flights of the Vedanta.
When the Vyadha finished his teaching, the Sannyasin felt astonished. He said, "Why are you in
that body? With such knowledge as yours why
are you in a Vyadha's body, and doing such
filthy, ugly work?" "My son," replied the Vyadha, "no duty is ugly, no duty is impure. My birth
placed me in these circumstances and environ-

ments. In my boyhood I learnt the trade; I am unattached and I try to do my duty well. I try to do my duty as a householder, and I try to do all I can to make my father and mother happy. I neither know your Yoga, nor have I become a Sannyasin, nor did I go out of the world into a forest; nevertheless, all that you have heard and seen has come to me through the unattached doing of the duty which belongs to my position."

There is a sage in India, a great Yogi, one of the most wonderful men I have ever seen in my life. He is a peculiar man, he will not teach anyone; if you ask him a question, he will not answer. It is too much for him to take up the position of a teacher, he will not do it. If you ask a question, and wait for some days, in the course of conversation he will bring up the subject, and wonderful light will he throw on it. He told me once the secret of work, "Let the end and the means be joined into one." When you are doing any work, do not think of anything beyond. Do it as worship, as the highest worship, and devote your whole life to it for the time being. Thus, in the story, the Vyadha and the woman did their duty with cheerfulness and whole-heartedness; and the result was that they became illuminated; clearly showing that the right performance of the duties of any station in life, without attachment to results, leads us to the highest realisation of the perfection of the soul.

It is the worker who is attached to results that grumbles about the nature of the duty which has fallen to his lot; to the unattached worker all duties are equally good and form efficient instruments with which selfishness and sensuality may be killed and the freedom of the soul secured. We are all apt to think too highly of ourselves. Our duties are determined by our deserts to a much larger extent than we are willing to grant. Competition rouses envy, and it kills the kindliness of the heart. To the grumbler all duties are distasteful; nothing will ever satisfy him, and his whole life is doomed to prove a failure. Let us work on, doing as we go whatever happens to be our duty and being ever ready to put our shoulders to the wheel. Then surely shall we see the Light!

WE HELP OURSELVES, NOT THE WORLD

BEFORE considering further how devotion to duty helps us in our spiritual progress, let me place before you in a brief compass another aspect of what we in India mean by Karma. In every religion there are three parts: philosophy, mythology, and ritual. Philosophy of course is the essence of every religion; mythology explains and illustrates it by means of the more or less legendary lives of great men, stories, and fables of wonderful things and so on; ritual gives to that philosophy a still more concrete form so that everyone may grasp it—ritual is, in fact, concretised philosophy. This ritual is Karma; it is necessary in every religion, because most of us cannot understand abstract spiritual things until we grow much spiritually. It is easy for men to think that they can understand anything, but when it comes to practical experience, they find that abstract ideas are often very hard to comprehend. Therefore symbols are of great help, and we cannot dispense with the symbolical method of putting things before us. From time immemorial symbols have been used by all kinds of religions. In one sense we cannot think but in symbols; words themselves are symbols of thought. In another sense everything in the universe may be looked upon as a symbol. The whole universe is a symbol, and God is the essence behind. This kind of symbology is not simply the creation of man; it is not that certain people belonging to a religion sit down together and think out certain symbols, and bring them into existence out of their own minds. The symbols of religion have a natural growth. Otherwise, why is it that certain symbols are associated with certain ideas in the mind of almost everyone? Certain symbols are universally prevalent. Many of you may think that the cross first came into existence as a symbol in connection with the Christian religion; but as a matter of fact, it existed before Christianity was, before Moses was born, before the Vedas were given out, before there was any human record of human things. The cross may be found to have been in existence among the Aztecs and the Phoenicians: every race seems to have had the cross. Again, the symbol of the crucified Saviour, of a man crucified upon a cross, appears to have been known to almost every nation. The circle has been a great symbol throughout the world. Then there is the most universal of all symbols, the Swastika. At one time it was thought that the Buddhists carried it all over the world with them, but it has been found out that ages before Buddhism it was used among nations. In old Babylon and in Egypt it was to be found. What does this show? All these symbols could not have been purely conventional. There must be some reason for them, some natural association between them and the human mind. Language is not the result of convention; it is not that people ever agreed to represent certain ideas by certain words; there never was an idea without a corresponding word or a word without a corresponding idea; ideas and words are in their nature inseparable. The symbols to represent ideas may be sound symbols or colour symbols. Deaf and dumb people have to think with other than sound symbols. Every thought in the mind has a form as its counterpart. This is called in Sanskrit philosophy Nâma-Rupa—name and form. It is as impossible to create by convention a system of symbols as it is to create a language. In the world's ritualistic symbols we have an expression of the religious thought of humanity. It is easy to say that there is no use of rituals and temples and all such paraphernalia; every baby says that in modern times. But it must be easy for all to see that those who worship inside a temple are in many respects different from those who will not worship there. Therefore the association of particular temples, rituals, and other concrete forms with particular religions has a tendency to bring into the mind of the followers of those religions the thoughts for which those concrete things stand as symbols; and it is not wise to ignore rituals and symbology altogether. The study and practice of these things form naturally a part of Karma-Yoga.

There are many other aspects of this science of work. One among them is to know the relation between thought and word and what can be achieved by the power of the word. In every religion the power of the word is recognised, so much so that in some of them creation itself is said to have come out of the word. The external aspect of the thought of God is the word, and as God thought and willed before He created, creation came out of the word. In this stress and hurry of our materialistic life our nerves lose sensibility and become hardened. The older we grow, the longer we are knocked about in the world, the more callous we become; and we are apt to neglect things that even happen persistently and prominently around us. Human nature, however, asserts itself sometimes, and we are led to inquire into and wonder at some of these common occurrences; wondering thus is the first step in the acquisition of light. Apart from the higher philosophic and religious value of the word, we may see that sound symbols play a prominent part in the drama of human life. I am talking to you. I am not touching you; the pulsations of the air caused by my speaking go into your ear, they touch your nerves and produce effects in your minds. You cannot resist this. What can be more wonderful than this? One man calls another a fool, and at this the other stands up and clenches his fist and lands a blow on his nose. Look at the power of the word! There is a woman weeping and miserable; another woman comes along and speaks to her a few gentle words; the doubled up frame of the weeping woman becomes straightened at once, her sorrow is gone and she already begins to smile. Think of the power of words! They are a great force in higher philosophy as well as in common life. Day and night we manipulate this force without thought and without inquiry. To know the nature of this force and to use it well is also a part of Karma-Yoga.

Our duty to others means helping others, doing good to the world. Why should we do good to the world? Apparently to help the world, but really to help ourselves. We should always try to help the world, that should be the highest motive in us; but if we consider well, we find that the world does not require our help at all. This world was not made that you or I should come and help it. I once read a sermon in which it was said: "All this beautiful world is very good, because it gives us time and opportunity to help others." Apparently this is a very beautiful sentiment, but is it not a blasphemy to say that the world needs our help? We cannot deny that there is much misery in it; to go out and help others is, therefore, the best thing we can do, although in the long run we shall find that helping others is only helping ourselves. As a boy I had some white mice. They were kept in a little box in which there were little wheels, and when the mice tried to cross the wheels, the wheels turned and turned, and the mice never got anywhere. So it is with the world and our helping it. The only help is that we get moral exercise. This world is neither good nor evil; each man manufactures a world for himself. If a blind man begins to think of the world, it is either as soft or hard, or as cold or hot. We are a mass of happiness or misery; we have seen that hundreds of times in our lives. As a rule the young are optimistic and the old pessimistic. The young have life before them; the old complain their day is gone; hundreds of desires, which they cannot fulfil, struggle in their hearts. Both are foolish nevertheless. Life is good or evil according to the state of mind in which we look at it, it is neither by itself. Fire, by itself, is neither good nor evil. When it

keeps us warm, we say "How beautiful is fire!"
When it burns our fingers, we blame it. Still, in
itself it is neither good nor bad. According as we
use it, it produces in us the feeling of good or
bad; so also is this world. It is perfect. By perfection is meant that it is perfectly fitted to meet
its ends. We may all be perfectly sure that it will
go on beautifully well without us, and we need
not bother our heads wishing to help it.

Yet we must do good; the desire to do good
is the highest motive power we have, if we
know all the time that it is a privilege to help
others. Do not stand on a high pedestal and
take five cents in your hand and say, "Here, my
poor man", but be grateful that the poor man
is there so that by making a gift to him you are
able to help yourself. It is not the receiver that
is blessed, but it is the giver. Be thankful that
you are allowed to exercise your power of
benevolence and mercy in the world, and thus
become pure and perfect. All good acts tend
to make us pure and perfect. What can we do
at best? Build a hospital, make roads, or erect
charity asylums! We may organise a charity and
collect two or three millions of dollars, build a
hospital with one million, with the second give
balls and drink champagne, and of the third let
the officers steal half, and leave the rest finally
to reach the poor; but what are all these? One

mighty wind in five minutes can break all your
buildings up. What shall we do then? One vol-
canic eruption may sweep away all our roads
and hospitals and cities and buildings. Let us
give up all this foolish talk of doing good to the
world. It is not waiting for your or my help; yet
we must work and constantly do good, because
it is a blessing to ourselves. That is the only way
we can become perfect. No beggar whom we
have helped has ever owed a single cent to us;
we owe everything to him, because he has
allowed us to exercise our charity on him. It is
entirely wrong to think that we have done or
can do good to the world, or to think that we
have helped such and such people. It is a foolish
thought, and all foolish thoughts bring misery.
We think that we have helped some man and
expect him to thank us; and because he does
not, unhappiness comes to us. Why should we
expect anything in return for what we do? Be
grateful to the man you help, think of him as
God. Is it not a great privilege to be allowed
to worship God by helping our fellow-men? If
we were really unattached, we should escape
all this pain of vain expectation, and could
cheerfully do good work in the world. Never
will unhappiness or misery come through work
done without attachment. The world will go on
with its happiness and misery through eternity.

There was a poor man who wanted some money; and somehow he had heard that if he could get hold of a ghost, he might command him to bring money or anything else he liked; so he was very anxious to get hold of a ghost. He went about searching for a man who would give him a ghost; and at last he found a sage, with great powers, and besought his help. The sage asked him what he would do with a ghost. "I want a ghost to work for me; teach me how to get hold of one, sir; I desire it very much", replied the man. But the sage said, "Don't disturb yourself, go home." The next day the man went again to the sage and began to weep and pray, "Give me a ghost; I must have a ghost, sir, to help me." At last the sage was disgusted, and said, "Take this charm, repeat this magic word, and a ghost will come, and whatever you say to him he will do. But beware; they are terrible beings, and must be kept continually busy. If you fail to give him work, he will take your life." The man replied, "That is easy; I can give him work for all his life." Then he went to a forest; and after long repetition of the magic word, a huge ghost appeared before him, and said, "I am a ghost. I have been conquered by your magic; but you must keep me constantly employed. The moment you fail to give me work I will kill you." The man said, "Build me a palace", and the ghost said, "It is done; the palace is built." "Bring me money", said the man. "Here is your money", said the ghost. "Cut this forest down, and build a city in its place." "That is done", said the ghost, "anything more?" Now the man began to be frightened and thought, "I can give him nothing more to do; he does everything in a trice." The ghost said, "Give me something to do or I will eat you up." The poor man could find no further occupation for him and was frightened. So he ran and ran and at last reached the sage and said, "O sir, protect my life!" The sage asked him what the matter was, and the man replied, "I have nothing to give the ghost to do. Everything I tell him to do he does in a moment, and he threatens to eat me up if I do not give him work." Just then the ghost arrived, saying, "I'll eat you up." And he would have swallowed the man. The man began to shake and begged the sage to save his life. The sage said, "I will find you a way out. Look at that dog with a curly tail. Draw your sword quickly and cut the tail off and give it to the ghost to straighten out." The man cut off the dog's tail and gave it to the ghost saying, "Straighten that out for me". The ghost took it and slowly and carefully straightened it out, but as soon as he let it go, it instantly curled up again. Once more he laboriously

straightened it out, only to find it again curled
up as soon as he attempted to let go of it. Again
he patiently straightened it out, but as soon as
he let it go, it curled up again. So he went on
for days and days, until he was exhausted and
said, "I was never in such trouble before in my
life. I am an old veteran ghost, but never before
was I in such trouble." "I will make a compro-
mise with you," he said to the man, "you let me
off, and I will let you keep all I have given
you and will promise not to harm you." The
man was much pleased and accepted the offer
gladly.

This world is like a dog's curly tail, and
people have been striving to straighten it out
for hundreds of years; but when they let it go,
it has curled up again. How could it be otherwise? One must first know how to work without
attachment, then one will not be a fanatic.
When we know that this world is like a dog's
curly tail and will never get straightened, we
shall not become fanatics. If there were no
fanaticism in the world, it would make much
more progress than it does now. It is a mistake
to think that fanaticism can make for the progress of mankind. On the contrary, it is a retard-
ing element creating hatred and anger, and
causing people to fight each other, and making
them unsympathetic. We think that whatever

we do or possess is the best in the world, and what we do not do or possess is of no value. So always remember the instance of the curly tail of the dog whenever you have a tendency to become a fanatic. You need not worry or make yourself sleepless about the world; it will go on without you. When you have avoided fanaticism, then alone will you work well. It is the level-headed man, the calm man, of good judgment and cool nerves, of great sympathy and love, who does good work and so does good to himself. The fanatic is foolish and has no sympathy; he can never straighten the world nor himself become pure and perfect.

To recapitulate the chief points in today's lecture: First, we have to bear in mind that we are all debtors to the world, and the world does not owe us anything. It is a great privilege for all of us to be allowed to do anything for the world. In helping the world we really help ourselves. The second point is that there is a God in this universe. It is not true that this universe is drifting and stands in need of help from you and me. God is ever present therein. He is undying and eternally active and infinitely watchful. When the whole universe sleeps, He sleeps not; He is working incessantly; all the changes and manifestations of the world are His. Thirdly, we ought not to hate anyone. This world will always continue to be a mixture of good and evil. Our duty is to sympathise with the weak and to love even the wrong-doer. The world is a grand moral gymnasium wherein we have all to take exercise so as to become stronger and stronger spiritually. Fourthly, we ought not to be fanatics of any kind, because fanaticism is opposed to love. You hear fanatics glibly saying, "I do not hate the sinner, I hate the sin"; but I am prepared to go any distance to see the face of that man who can really make a distinction between the sin and the sinner. It is easy to say so. If we can distinguish well between quality and substance, we may become perfect men. It is not easy to do this. And further, the calmer we are and the less disturbed our nerves, the more shall we love and the better will our work be.

NON-ATTACHMENT IS COMPLETE
SELF-ABNEGATION

JUST as every action that emanates from us comes back to us as reaction, even so our actions may act on other people and theirs on us. Perhaps all of you have observed it as a fact that when persons do evil actions, they become more and more evil, and when they begin to do good, they become stronger and stronger and learn to do good at all times. This intensification of the influence of action cannot be explained on any other ground than that we can act and react upon each other. To take an illustration from physical science, when I am doing a certain action, my mind may be said to be in a certain state of vibration; all minds which are in similar circumstances will have the tendency to be affected by my mind. If there are different musical instruments tuned alike in one room, all of you may have noticed that when one is struck, the others have the tendency to vibrate so as to give the same note. So all minds that have the same tension, so to say, will be equally affected by the same thought. Of course this influence of thought on mind will vary according to distance and other causes, but the mind is always open to affection. Suppose I am doing an evil act, my mind is in a certain state of vibration, and all minds in the universe, which are in a similar state, have the possibility of being affected by the vibration of my mind. So when I am doing a good action, my mind is in another state of vibration; and all minds similarly strung have the possibility of being affected by my mind; and this power of mind upon mind is more or less according as the force of the tension is greater or less.

Following this simile further, it is quite possible that, just as light waves may travel for millions of years before they reach any object, so thought waves may also travel hundreds of years before they meet an object with which they vibrate in unison. It is quite possible, therefore, that this atmosphere of ours is full of such thought pulsations, both good and evil. Every thought projected from every brain goes on pulsating, as it were, until it meets a fit object that will receive it. Any mind which is open to receive some of these impulses will take them immediately. So when a man is doing evil actions, he has brought his mind to a certain state of tension, and all the waves which correspond to that state of tension and which may be said to be already in the atmosphere, will struggle to enter into his mind. That is why an evildoer generally goes on doing more and more evil. His actions become intensified. Such also will be the case with the doer of good; he will open himself to all the good waves that are in the atmosphere, and his good actions also will become intensified. We run, therefore, a twofold danger in doing evil: first, we open ourselves to all the evil influences surrounding us; secondly, we create evil which affects others, may be hundreds of years hence. In doing evil we injure ourselves and others also. In doing good we do good to ourselves and to others as well; and like all other forces in man, these forces of good and evil also gather strength from outside.

According to Karma-Yoga, the action one has done cannot be destroyed until it has borne its fruit; no power in nature can stop it from yielding its results. If I do an evil action, I must suffer for it; there is no power in this universe to stop or stay it. Similarly if I do a good action, there is no power in the universe which can stop its bearing good results. The cause must have its effect; nothing can prevent or restrain this. Now comes a very fine and serious question about Karma-Yoga—namely, that these actions of ours, both good and evil, are intimately connected with each other. We cannot put a line of demarcation, and say this action is entirely good and this entirely evil. There is no action which does not bear good and evil fruits at the

same time. To take the nearest example: I am
talking to you, and some of you, perhaps, think
I am doing good and at the same time I am,
perhaps, killing thousands of microbes in the
atmosphere; I am thus doing evil to something
else. When it is very near to us and affects those
we know, we say that it is very good action if
it affects them in a good manner. For instance,
you may call my speaking to you very good, but
the microbes will not; the microbes you do not
see, but yourselves you do see. The way in
which my talk affects you is obvious to you, but
how it affects the microbes is not so obvious.
And so, if we analyse our evil actions also, we
may find that some good possibly results from
them somewhere. He who in good action sees
that there is something evil in it, and in the
midst of evil sees that there is something
good in it somewhere—has known the secret
of work.

But what follows from it? That, howsoever
we may try, there cannot be any action which is
perfectly pure or any which is perfectly impure,
taking purity and impurity in the sense of injury
and non-injury. We cannot breathe or live without injuring others, and every bit of the food we
eat is taken away from another's mouth. Our very
lives are crowding out other lives. It may be
men or animals or small microbes, but some one

or other of these we have to crowd out. That being the case, it naturally follows that perfection can never be attained by work. We may work through all eternity, but there will be no way out of this intricate maze; you may work on, and on, and on; there will be no end to this inevitable association of good and evil in the results of work.

The second point to consider is, what is the end of work? We find the vast majority of people in every country believing that there will be a time when this world will become perfect, when there will be no disease, nor death nor unhappiness nor wickedness. That is a very good idea, a very good motive power to inspire and uplift the ignorant; but if we think for a moment, we shall find on the very face of it that it cannot be so. How can it be, seeing that good and evil are the obverse and reverse of the same coin? How can you have good without evil at the same time? What is meant by perfection? A perfect life is a contradiction in terms. Life itself is a state of continuous struggle between ourselves and everything outside. Every moment we are fighting actually with external nature, and if we are defeated, our life has to go. It is, for instance, a continuous struggle for food and air. If food or air fails, we die. Life is not a simple and smoothly flowing thing, but it is a compound effect. This complex struggle between something inside and the external world is what we call life. So it is clear that when this struggle ceases, there will be an end of life.

What is meant by ideal happiness is the cessation of this struggle. But then life will cease, for the struggle can only cease when life itself has ceased. We have seen already that in helping the world we help ourselves. The main effect of work done for others is to purify ourselves. By means of the constant effort to do good to others we are trying to forget ourselves; this forgetfulness of self is the one great lesson we have to learn in life. Man thinks foolishly that he can make himself happy, and after years of struggle finds out at last that true happiness consists in killing selfishness and that no one can make him happy except himself. Every act of charity, every thought of sympathy, every action of help, every good deed, is taking so much of self-importance away from our little selves and making us think of ourselves as the lowest and the least; and, therefore, it is all good. Here we find that Jnana, Bhakti, and Karma all come to one point. The highest ideal is eternal and entire self-abnegation, where there is no "I", but all is "Thou"; and whether he is conscious or unconscious of it, Karma-Yoga leads man to that end. A religious preacher may become horrified at the idea of an Impersonal God; he may insist on a Personal God and wish to keep up his own identity and individuality, whatever he may mean by that. But his ideas of ethics, if they are really good, cannot but be based on the highest self-abnegation. It is the basis of all morality; you may extend it to men or animals or angels, it is the one basic idea, the one fundamental principle running through all ethical systems.

You will find various classes of men in this world. First, there are the God-men whose self-abnegation is complete and who do only good to others even at the sacrifice of their own lives. These are the highest of men. If there are a hundred of such in any country, that country need never despair. But they are unfortunately too few. Then there are the good men who do good to others so long as it does not injure themselves. And there is a third class who, to do good to themselves, injure others. It is said by a Sanskrit poet that there is a fourth unnamable class of people who injure others merely for injury's sake. Just as there are at one pole of existence the highest good men who do good for the sake of doing good, so at the other pole, there are others who injure others just for the sake of the injury. They do not gain anything thereby, but it is their nature to do evil.

Here are two Sanskrit words. The one is Pravritti which means revolving towards, and the other is Nivritti which means revolving away. The "revolving towards" is what we call the world, the "I and mine"; it includes all those things which are always enriching that "me" by wealth and money and power, and name and fame, and which are of a grasping nature, always tending to accumulate everything in one centre, that centre being "myself". That is the Pravritti, the natural tendency of every human being; taking everything from everywhere and heaping it around one centre, that centre being man's own sweet self. When this tendency begins to break, when it is Nivritti or going away from, then begin morality and religion. Both Pravritti and Nivritti are of the nature of work; the former is evil work, and the latter is good work. This Nivritti is the fundamental basis of all morality and all religion, and the very perfection of it is entire self-abnegation, readiness to sacrifice mind and body and everything for another being. When a man has reached that state, he has attained to the perfection of Karma-Yoga. This is the highest result of good works. Although a man has not studied a single system of philosophy, although he does not believe in any God and never has believed, although he has not prayed even once in his whole life, if

the simple power of good actions has brought
him to that state where he is ready to give up
his life and all else for others, he has arrived at
the same point to which the religious man will
come through his prayers and the philosopher
through his knowledge; and so you may find that
the philosopher, the worker, and the devotee, all
meet at one point, that one point being self-
abnegation. However much their systems of
philosophy and religion may differ, all mankind
stand in reverence and awe before the man who
is ready to sacrifice himself for others. Here it is
not at all any question of creed or doctrine—
even men who are very much opposed to all
religious ideas, when they see one of these acts
of complete self-sacrifice, feel that they must
revere it. Have you not seen even a most bigoted
Christian, when he reads Edwin Arnold's *Light
of Asia*, stand in reverence of Buddha who
preached no God, preached nothing but self-
sacrifice? The only thing is that the bigot does
not know that his own end and aim in life is
exactly the same as that of those from whom he
differs. The worshipper, by keeping constantly
before him the idea of God and a surrounding
of good, comes to the same point at last and says,
"Thy will be done", and keeps nothing to himself. That is self-abnegation. The philosopher,
with his knowledge, sees that the seeming self

is a delusion and easily gives it up. It is self-abnegation. So Karma, Bhakti, and Jnana all meet here; and this is what was meant by all the great preachers of ancient times when they taught that God is not the world. There is one thing which is the world and another which is God; and this distinction is very true; what they mean by world is selfishness. Unselfishness is God. One may live on a throne in a golden palace and be perfectly unselfish; and then he is in God. Another may live in a hut and wear rags and have nothing in the world; yet, if he is selfish, he is intensely merged in the world.

To come back to one of our main points, we say that we cannot do good without at the same time doing some evil, or do evil without doing some good. Knowing this, how can we work? There have, therefore, been sects in this world who have in an astoundingly preposterous way preached slow suicide as the only means to get out of the world because, if a man lives, he has to kill poor little animals and plants or do injury to something or some one. So, according to them, the only way out of the world is to die. The Jainas have preached this doctrine as their highest ideal. This teaching seems to be very logical. But the true solution is found in the Gita. It is the theory of non-attachment, to be attached to nothing while doing our work of

life. Know that you are separated entirely from
the world though you are in the world, and that
whatever you may be doing in it, you are not
doing that for your own sake. Any action that
you do for yourself will bring its effect to bear
upon you. If it is a good action, you will have
to take the good effect, and if bad, you will have
to take the bad effect; but any action that is
not done for your own sake, whatever it be, will
have no effect on you. There is to be found
a very expressive sentence in our scriptures
embodying this idea: "Even if he kill the whole
universe (or be himself killed), he is neither the
killer nor the killed, when he knows that he is not
acting for himself at all." Therefore Karma-Yoga
teaches, "Do not give up the world; live in the
world, imbibe its influences as much as you can;
but if it be for your own enjoyment's sake, work
not at all." Enjoyment should not be the goal.
First kill your self and then take the whole
world as yourself; as the old Christians used to
say, "The old man must die." This old man is
the selfish idea that the whole world is made for
our enjoyment. Foolish parents teach their
children to pray, "O Lord, Thou hast created
this sun for me and this moon for me", as if the
Lord has had nothing else to do than to create
everything for these babies. Do not teach your
children such nonsense. Then again, there are

people who are foolish in another way; they teach us that all these animals were created for us to kill and eat, and that this universe is for the enjoyment of men. That is all foolishness. A tiger may say, "Man was created for me", and pray, "O Lord, how wicked are these men who do not come and place themselves before me to be eaten; they are breaking Your law." If the world is created for us, we are also created for the world. That this world is created for our enjoyment is the most wicked idea that holds us down. This world is not for our sake. Millions pass out of it every year; the world does not feel it; millions of others are supplied in their place. Just as much as the world is for us, so we also are for the world.

To work properly, therefore, you have first to give up the idea of attachment. Secondly, do not mix in the fray, hold yourself as a witness and go on working. My Master used to say, "Look upon your children as a nurse does." The nurse will take your baby and fondle it and play with it and behave towards it as gently as if it were her own child; but as soon as you give her notice to quit, she is ready to start off bag and baggage from the house. Everything in the shape of attachment is forgotten; it will not give the ordinary nurse the least pang to leave your children and take up other children. Even so are

you to be with all that you consider your own.
You are the nurse, and if you believe in God,
believe that all these things which you consider
yours are really His. The greatest weakness
often insinuates itself as the greatest good and
strength. It is a weakness to think that anyone
is dependent on me, and that I can do good to
another. This belief is the mother of all our
attachment, and through this attachment comes
all our pain. We must inform our minds that
no one in this universe depends upon us; not one
beggar depends on our charity; not one soul on
our kindness; not one living thing on our help.
All are helped on by nature, and will be so
helped even though millions of us were not
here. The course of nature will not stop for such
as you and me; it is, as already pointed out, only
a blessed privilege to you and to me that we
are allowed, in the way of helping others, to
educate ourselves. This is a great lesson to learn
in life; and when we have learnt it fully, we
shall never be unhappy; we can go and mix
without harm in society anywhere and everywhere. You may have wives and husbands, and
regiments of servants, and kingdoms to govern;
if only you act on the principle that the world
is not for you and does not inevitably need you,
they can do you no harm. This very year some
of your friends may have died. Is the world

waiting without going on for them to come again? Is its current stopped? No, it goes on. So drive out of your mind the idea that you have to do something for the world; the world does not require any help from you. It is sheer nonsense on the part of any man to think that he is born to help the world; it is simply pride, it is selfishness insinuating itself in the form of virtue. When you have trained your mind and your nerves to realise this idea of the world's non-dependence on you or on anybody, there will then be no reaction in the form of pain resulting from work. When you give something to a man and expect nothing—do not even expect the man to be grateful—his ingratitude will not tell upon you, because you never expected anything, never thought you had any right to anything in the way of a return; you gave him what he deserved; his own Karma got it for him; your Karma made you the carrier thereof. Why should you be proud of having given away something? You are the porter that carried the money or other kind of gift, and the world deserved it by its own Karma. Where is then the reason for pride in you? There is nothing very great in what you give to the world. When you have acquired the feeling of non-attachment, there will then be neither good nor evil for you. It is only selfishness that causes the difference between good and evil. It is a very hard thing to understand, but you will come to learn in time that nothing in the universe has power over you until you allow it to exercise such a power. Nothing has power over the Self of man, until the Self becomes a fool and loses independence. So by non-attachment you overcome and deny the power of anything to act upon you. It is very easy to say that nothing has the right to act upon you until you allow it to do so; but what is the true sign of the man who really does not allow anything to work upon him, who is neither happy nor unhappy when acted upon by the external world? The sign is that good or ill fortune causes no change in his mind; in all conditions he continues to remain the same.

There was a great sage in India called Vyâsa. This Vyasa is known as the author of the Vedanta aphorisms, and was a holy man. His father had tried to become a very perfect man and had failed. His grandfather had also tried and failed. His great-grandfather had similarly tried and failed. He himself did not succeed perfectly, but his son, Shuka, was born perfect. Vyasa taught his son wisdom; and after teaching him the knowledge of truth himself, he sent him to the court of King Janaka. He was a great king and was called Janaka Videha. Videha means "without a body". Although a king, he had

entirely forgotten that he was a body; he felt
that he was a spirit all the time. This boy Shuka
was sent to be taught by him. The king knew
that Vyasa's son was coming to him to learn
wisdom; so he made certain arrangements
beforehand; and when the boy presented himself at the gates of the palace, the guards took
no notice of him whatsoever. They only gave
him a seat, and he sat there for three days and
nights, nobody speaking to him, nobody asking
him who he was or whence he was. He was
the son of a very great sage; his father was
honoured by the whole country, and he himself
was a most respectable person; yet the low,
vulgar guards of the palace would take no notice
of him. After that, suddenly, the ministers of the
king and all the big officials came there and received him with the greatest honours. They
conducted him in and showed him into splendid
rooms, gave him the most fragrant baths and
wonderful dresses, and for eight days they kept
him there in all kinds of luxury. That solemnly
serene face of Shuka did not change even to the
smallest extent by the change in the treatment
accorded to him; he was the same in the midst
of this luxury as when waiting at the door. Then
he was brought before the king. The king was
on his throne, music was playing, and dancing
and other amusements were going on. The king

KY-7

then gave him a cup of milk, full to the brim, and asked him to go seven times round the hall without spilling even a drop. The boy took the cup and proceeded in the midst of the music and the attraction of the beautiful faces. As desired by the king, seven times did he go round, and not a drop of the milk was spilt. The boy's mind could not be attracted by anything in the world, unless he allowed it to affect him. And when he brought the cup to the king, the king said to him, "What your father has taught you and what you have learnt yourself, I can only repeat; you have known the truth; go home."

Thus the man that has practised control over himself cannot be acted upon by anything outside; there is no more slavery for him. His mind has become free; such a man alone is fit to live well in the world. We generally find men holding two opinions regarding the world. Some are pessimists and say, "How horrible this world is, how wicked!" Some others are optimists and say, "How beautiful this world is, how wonderful!" To those who have not controlled their own minds, the world is either full of evil or at best a mixture of good and evil. This very world will become to us an optimistic world when we become masters of our own minds. Nothing will then work upon us as good or evil; we shall find everything to be in its proper place, to be harmonious. Some men, who begin by saying that the world is a hell, often end by saying that it is a heaven when they succeed in the practice of self-control. If we are genuine Karma-Yogis and wish to train ourselves to the attainment of this state, wherever we may begin we are sure to end in perfect self-abnegation; and as soon as this seeming self has gone, the whole world, which at first appears to us to be filled with evil, will appear to be heaven itself and full of blessedness. Its very atmosphere will be blessed; every human face there will be good. Such is the end and aim of Karma-Yoga, and such is its perfection in practical life.

Our various Yogas do not conflict with each other; each of them leads us to the same goal and makes us perfect; only each has to be strenuously practised. The whole secret is in practising. First you have to hear, then think, and then practise. This is true of every Yoga. You have first to hear about it and understand what it is; and many things which you do not understand will be made clear to you by constant hearing and thinking. It is hard to understand everything at once. The explanation of everything is after all in yourself. No one was ever really taught by another; each of us has to teach himself. The external teacher offers only

the suggestion which rouses the internal teacher
to work to understand things. Then things will
be made clearer to us by our own power of per-
ception and thought, and we shall realise them
in our own souls; and that realisation will grow
into the intense power of will. First it is feeling,
then it becomes willing, and out of that willing
comes the tremendous force for work that will
go through every vein and nerve and muscle,
until the whole mass of your body is changed
into an instrument of the unselfish Yoga of work,
and the desired result of perfect self-abnegation and utter unselfishness is duly attained. This
attainment does not depend on any dogma or
doctrine or belief. Whether one is Christian or
Jew or Gentile, it does not matter. Are you unselfish? That is the question. If you are, you will
be perfect without reading a single religious
book, without going into a single church or
temple. Each one of our Yogas is fitted to make
man perfect even without the help of the others,
because they have all the same goal in view.
The Yogas of work, of wisdom, and of devotion
are all capable of serving as direct and indepen-
dent means for the attainment of Moksha. "Fools
alone say that work and philosophy are different,
not the learned." The learned know that, though
apparently different from each other, they at
last lead to the same goal of human perfection.

FREEDOM

In addition to meaning work, we have stated that psychologically the word Karma also implies causation. Any work, any action, any thought that produces an effect is called a Karma. Thus the law of Karma means the law of causation, of inevitable cause and sequence. Wheresoever there is a cause, there an effect must be produced; this necessity cannot be resisted, and this law of Karma, according to our philosophy, is true throughout the whole universe. Whatever we see or feel or do, whatever action there is anywhere in the universe, while being the effect of past work on the one hand, becomes, on the other, a cause in its turn and produces its own effect. It is necessary, together with this, to consider what is meant by the word "law". By law is meant the tendency of a series to repeat itself. When we see one event followed by another, or sometimes happening simultaneously with another, we expect this sequence or co-existence to recur. Our old logicians and philosophers of the Nyâya school call this law by the name of Vyâpti. According to them all our ideas of law are due to association. A series of phenomena becomes associated with things in our mind in a sort of invariable order, so that whatever we perceive at any time is immediately referred to other facts in the mind. Any one idea or, according to our psychology, any one wave that is produced in the mind-stuff, Chitta, must always give rise to many similar waves. This is the psychological idea of association, and causation is only an aspect of this grand, pervasive principle of association. This pervasiveness of association is what is called, in Sanskrit, Vyâpti. In the external world the idea of law is the same as in the internal—the expectation that a particular phenomenon will be followed by another, and that the series will repeat itself. Really speaking, therefore, law does not exist in nature. Practically it is an error to say that gravitation exists in the earth, or that there is any law existing objectively anywhere in nature. Law is the method, the manner in which our mind grasps a series of phenomena; it is all in the mind. Certain phenomena, happening one after another or together, and followed by the conviction of the regularity of their recurrence, thus enabling our minds to grasp the method of the whole series, constitute what we call law.

The next question for consideration is what we mean by law being universal. Our universe is that portion of existence which is characterised by what the Sanskrit psychologists call Desha-Kâla-Nimitta, or what is known to European psychology as space, time, and causation. This universe is only a part of infinite existence thrown into a peculiar mould, composed of space, time, and causation. It necessarily follows that law is possible only within this conditioned universe; beyond it there cannot be any law. When we speak of the universe, we only mean that portion of existence which is limited by our mind—the universe of the senses, which we can see, feel, touch, hear, think of, imagine. This alone is under law; but beyond it, existence cannot be subject to law, because causation does not extend beyond the world of our minds. Anything beyond the range of our mind and our senses is not bound by the law of causation, as there is no mental association of things in the region beyond the senses, and no causation without association of ideas. It is only when "being" or existence gets moulded into name and form that it obeys the law of causation and is said to be under law, because all law has its essence in causation. Therefore we see at once that there cannot be any such thing as free will; the very words are a contradiction, because will is what we know, and everything that we know is within our universe, and everything within our universe is moulded by the conditions of space, time, and causation. Everything that we know, or can possibly know, must be subject to causation, and that which obeys the law of causation cannot be free. It is acted upon by other agents and becomes a cause in its turn. But that which has become converted into the will, which was not the will before, but which, when it fell into this mould of space, time, and causation, became converted into the human will, is free; and when this will gets out of this mould of space, time, and causation, it will be free again. From freedom it comes and becomes moulded into this bondage, and it gets out and goes back to freedom again.

The question has been raised as to from whom this universe comes, in whom it rests, and to whom it goes; and the answer has been given that from freedom it comes, in bondage it rests, and goes back into that freedom again. So when we speak of man as no other than that infinite being which is manifesting itself, we mean that only one very small part thereof is man; this body and this mind which we see are only one part of the whole, only one spot of the infinite being. This whole universe is only one speck of the infinite being; and all our laws, our bondages, our joys and our sorrows, our happinesses and our expectations, are only within this small universe; all our progression and digression are within its small compass. So you see how childish it is to expect a continuation of this universe—the creation of our minds —and to expect to go to heaven, which after all must mean only a repetition of this world that we know. You see at once that it is an impossible and childish desire to make the whole of infinite existence conform to the limited and conditioned existence which we know. When a man says that he will have again and again this same thing which he is having now, or, as I sometimes put it, when he asks for a *comfortable* religion, you may know that he has become so degenerate that he cannot think of anything higher than what he is now; he is just his little present surroundings and nothing more. He has forgotten his infinite nature, and his whole idea is confined to these little joys and sorrows and heart-jealousies of the moment. He thinks that this finite thing is the infinite; and not only so, he will not let this foolishness go. He clings on desperately unto Trishnâ, the thirst after life, what the Buddhists call Tanhâ and Trissâ. There may be millions of kinds of happiness and beings and laws and progress and causation, all acting outside the little universe that we know, and, after all, the whole of this comprises but one section of our infinite nature.

To acquire freedom we have to get beyond the limitations of this universe; it cannot be found here. Perfect equilibrium, or what the Christians

call the peace that passeth all understanding,
cannot be had in this universe, nor in heaven,
nor in any place where our mind and thoughts
can go, where the senses can feel, or which the
imagination can conceive. No such place can
give us that freedom, because all such places
would be within our universe, and it is limited
by space, time, and causation. There may be
places that are more ethereal than this earth of
ours, where enjoyments may be keener, but even
those places must be in the universe and, therefore, in bondage to law; so we have to go
beyond, and real religion begins where this little
universe ends. These little joys and sorrows and
knowledge of things end there, and the reality
begins. Until we give up the thirst after life, the
strong attachment to this our transient, conditioned existence, we have no hope of catching
even a glimpse of that infinite freedom beyond.
It stands to reason then that there is only one
way to attain to the freedom which is the goal
of all the noblest aspirations of mankind, and
that is by giving up this little life, giving up
this little universe, giving up this earth, giving
up heaven, giving up the body, giving up the
mind, giving up everything that is limited and
conditioned. If we give up our attachment to
this little universe of the senses or of the mind,
we shall be free immediately. The only way to

come out of bondage is to go beyond the limitations of law, to go beyond causation.

But it is a most difficult thing to give up the clinging to this universe; few ever attain to that. These are two ways to do that, mentioned in our books. One is called the "Neti, Neti" (not this, not this), the other is called the "Iti" (this); the former is the negative, and the latter is the positive way. The negative way is the most difficult. It is only possible to the men of the very highest, exceptional minds and gigantic wills who simply stand up and say, "No, I will not have this", and the mind and body obey their will, and they come out successful. But such people are very rare. The vast majority of mankind choose the positive way, the way through the world, making use of all the bondages themselves to break those very bondages. This is also a kind of giving up; only it is done slowly and gradually, by knowing things, enjoying things, and thus obtaining experience, and knowing the nature of things until the mind lets them all go at last and becomes unattached. The former way of obtaining non-attachment is by reasoning, and the latter way is through work and experience. The first is the path of Jnana-Yoga and is characterised by the refusal to do any work; the second is that of Karma-Yoga in which there is no cessation from work. Everyone must work in the universe. Only those who are perfectly satisfied with the Self, whose desires do not go beyond the Self, whose mind never strays out of the Self, to whom the Self is all in all, only those do not work. The rest must work. A current rushing down of its own nature falls into a hollow and makes a whirlpool, and after running a little in that whirlpool, it emerges again in the form of the free current to go on unchecked. Each human life is like that current. It gets into the whirl, gets involved in this world of space, time, and causation, whirls round a little, crying out "my father, my brother, my name, my fame", and so on, and at last emerges out of it and regains its original freedom. The whole universe is doing that. Whether we know it or not, whether we are conscious or unconscious of it, we are all working to get out of the dream of the world of work. Man's experience in the world is to enable him to get out of its whirlpool.

What is Karma-Yoga? The knowledge of the secret of work. We see that the whole universe is working. For what? For salvation, for liberty; from the atom to the highest being working for the one end—liberty for the mind, for the body, for the spirit. All things are always trying to get freedom, flying away from bondage. The sun, the moon, the earth, the planets, all are trying to fly away from bondage. The centrifugal and the

centripetal forces of nature are indeed typical of
our universe. Instead of being knocked about in
this universe, and after long delay and thrashing,
getting to know things as they are, we learn from
Karma-Yoga the secret of work, the method of
work, the organising power of work. A vast mass
of energy may be spent in vain if we do not
know how to utilise it. Karma-Yoga makes a
science of work; you learn by it how best to
utilise all the workings of this world. Work is
inevitable, it must be so; but we should work
to the highest purpose. Karma-Yoga makes us
admit that this world is a world of five minutes;
that it is a something we have to pass through;
and that freedom is not here, but is only to be
found beyond. To find the way out of the bondages of the world we have to go through it
slowly and surely. There may be those exceptional persons about whom I just spoke, those
who can stand aside and give up the world as a
snake casts off its skin and stands aside and
looks at it. There are no doubt these exceptional
beings; but the rest of mankind have to go
slowly through the world of work. Karma-Yoga
shows the process, the secret, and the method
of doing it to the best advantage.

What does it say? "Work incessantly, but give
up all attachment to work." Do not identify
yourself with anything. Hold your mind free. All

this that you see, the pains and the miseries, are but the necessary conditions of this world; poverty and wealth and happiness are but momentary; they do not belong to our real nature at all. Our nature is far beyond misery and happiness, beyond every object of the senses, beyond the imagination; and yet we must go on working all the time. "Misery comes through attachment, not through work." As soon as we identify ourselves with the work we do, we feel miserable; but if we do not identify ourselves with it, we do not feel that misery. If a beautiful picture belonging to another is burnt, a man does not generally become miserable, but when his own picture is burnt, how miserable he feels! Why? Both were beautiful pictures, perhaps copies of the same original; but in one case very much more misery is felt than in the other. It is because in one case he identifies himself with the picture, and not in the other. This "I and mine" causes the whole misery. With the sense of possession comes selfishness, and selfishness, brings on misery. Every act of selfishness or thought of selfishness makes us attached to something, and immediately we are made slaves. Each wave in the Chitta that says "I and mine" immediately puts a chain round us and makes us slaves; and the more we say "I and mine", the more slavery grows, the more misery increases. Therefore

Karma-Yoga tells us to enjoy the beauty of all the pictures in the world, but not to identify ourselves with any of them. Never say "mine". Whenever we say a thing is mine, misery will immediately come. Do not even say "my child" in your mind. Possess the child, but do not say "mine". If you do, then will come the misery. Do not say "my house", do not say "my body". The whole difficulty is there. The body is neither yours nor mine, nor anybody's. These bodies are coming and going by the laws of nature, but we are free, standing as witness. This body is no more free than a picture or a wall. Why should we be attached so much to a body? If somebody paints a picture, he does it and passes on. Do not project that tentacle of selfishness, "I must possess it." As soon as that is projected, misery will begin.

So Karma-Yoga says, first destroy the tendency to project this tentacle of selfishness; and when you have the power of checking it, hold it in and do not allow the mind to get into the ways of selfishness. Then you may go out into the world and work as much you can. Mix everywhere, go where you please; you will never be contaminated with evil. There is the lotus leaf in the water; the water cannot touch and adhere to it; so will you be in the world. This is called Vairâgya, dispassion or non-attachment. I believe

I have told you that without non-attachment
there cannot be any kind of Yoga. Non-attachment is the basis of all the Yogas. The man who
gives up living in houses, wearing fine clothes,
and eating good food, and goes into the desert,
may be a most attached person. His only possession, his own body, may become everything
to him; and as he lives he will be simply struggling for the sake of his body. Non-attachment
does not mean anything that we may do in relation to our external body, it is all in the mind.
The binding link of "I and mine" is in the mind.
If we have not this link with the body and with
the things of the senses, we are non-attached,
wherever and whatever we may be. A man may
be on a throne and perfectly non-attached;
another man may be in rags and still very much
attached. First we have to attain this state of
non-attachment, and then to work incessantly.
Karma-Yoga gives us the method that will help
us in giving up all attachment, though it is
indeed very hard.

Here are the two ways of giving up all attachment. The one is for those who do not believe
in God, or in any outside help. They are left to
their own devices; they have simply to work with
their own will, with the powers of their mind
and discrimination, saying, "I must be non-
attached". For those who believe in God there

is another way, which is much less difficult. They give up the fruits of work unto the Lord, they work and are never attached to the results. Whatever they see, feel, hear, or do, is for Him. For whatever good work we may do, let us not claim any praise or benefit. It is the Lord's; give up the fruits unto Him. Let us stand aside and think that we are only servants obeying the Lord, our Master, and that every ·impulse for action comes from Him every moment. Whatever thou worshippest, whatever thou perceivest, whatever thou doest, give up all unto Him and be at rest. Let us be at peace, perfect peace, with ourselves, and give up our whole body and mind and everything as an eternal sacrifice unto the Lord. Instead of the sacrifice of pouring oblations into the fire, perform this one great sacrifice day and night—the sacrifice of your little self. "In search of wealth in this world, Thou art the only wealth I have found; I sacrifice myself unto Thee. In search of some one to be loved, Thou art the only one beloved I have found; I sacrifice myself unto Thee." Let us repeat this day and night, and say, "Nothing for me; no matter whether the thing is good, bad or indifferent; I do not care for it; I sacrifice all unto Thee." Day and night let us renounce our seeming self until it becomes a habit with us to do so, until it gets into the blood, the nerves, and the brain, and the whole body is every moment obedient to this idea of self-renunciation. Go then into the midst of the battlefield, with the roaring cannon and the din of war, and you will find yourself to be free and at peace.

Karma-Yoga teaches us that the ordinary idea of duty is on the lower plane; nevertheless, all of us have to do our duty. Yet we may see that this peculiar sense of duty is very often a great cause of misery. Duty becomes a disease with us; it drags us ever forward. It catches hold of us and makes our whole life miserable. It is the bane of human life. This duty, this idea of duty is the midday summer sun which scorches the innermost soul of mankind. Look at those poor slaves to duty! Duty leaves them no time to say prayers, no time to bathe. Duty is ever on them! They go out and work. Duty is on them! They come home and think of the work for the next day. Duty is on them! It is living a slave's life, at last dropping down in the street and dying in harness like a horse. This is duty as it is understood. The only true duty is to be unattached and to work as free beings, to give up all work unto God. All our duties are His. Blessed are we that we are ordered out here. We serve our time; whether we do it ill or well, who knows? If we do it well, we do not get the fruits.

If we do it ill, neither do we get the care. Be at rest, be free, and work. This kind of freedom is a very hard thing to attain. How easy it is to interpret slavery as duty—the morbid attachment of flesh for flesh as duty! Men go out into the world and struggle and fight for money or for any other thing to which they get attached. Ask them why they do it. They say, "It is a duty". It is the absurd greed for gold and gain, and they try to cover it with a few flowers.

What is duty after all? It is really the impulsion of the flesh, of our attachment; and when an attachment has become established, we call it duty. For instance, in countries where there is no marriage, there is no duty between husband and wife, when marriage comes, husband and wife live together on account of attachment; and that kind of living together becomes settled after generations; and when it becomes so settled, it becomes a duty. It is, so to say, a sort of chronic disease. When it is acute, we call it disease, when it is chronic, we call it nature. It is a disease. So when attachment becomes chronic, we baptise it with the high-sounding name of duty. We strew flowers upon it, trumpets sound for it, sacred texts are said over it, and then the whole world fights, and men earnestly rob each other for this duty's sake. Duty is good to the extent that it checks brutality. To the lowest kinds of men,

who cannot have any other ideal, it is of some
good; but those who want to be Karma-Yogis
must throw this idea of duty overboard. There is
no duty for you and me. Whatever you have to
give to the world, do give by all means, but not
as a duty. Do not take any thought of that. Be
not compelled. Why should you be compelled?
*Everything that you do under compulsion goes
to build up attachment.* Why should you have
any duty?

Resign everything unto God. In this tremendous fiery furnace where the fire of duty
scorches everybody, drink this cup of nectar and
be happy. We are all simply working out His
will, and have nothing to do with rewards and
punishments. If you want the reward, you must
also have the punishment; the only way to get
out of the punishment is to give up the reward.
The only way of getting out of misery is by
giving up the idea of happiness, because these
two are linked to each other. On one side there
is happiness, on the other there is misery. On
one side there is life, on the other there is death.
The only way to get beyond death is to give up
the love of life. Life and death are the same
thing, looked at from different points. So the
idea of happiness without misery or of life without death is very good for schoolboys and
children; but the thinker sees that it is all a con-

tradiction in terms and gives up both. Seek no praise, no reward for anything you do. No sooner do we perform a good action than we begin to desire credit for it. No sooner do we give money to some charity than we want to see our names blazoned in the papers. Misery must come as the result of such desires. The greatest men in the world have passed away unknown. The Buddhas and the Christs that we know are but second-rate heroes in comparison with the greatest men of whom the world knows nothing. Hundreds of these unknown heroes have lived in every country working silently. Silently they live and silently they pass away; and in time their thoughts find expression in Buddhas or Christs, and it is these latter that become known to us. The highest men do not seek to get any name or fame from their knowledge. They leave their ideas to the world; they put forth no claims for themselves and establish no schools or systems in their name. Their whole nature shrinks from such a thing. They are the pure Sâttvikas, who can never make any stir, but only melt down in love. I have seen one such Yogi who lives in a cave in India. He is one of the most wonderful men I have ever seen. He has so completely lost the sense of his own individuality that we may say that the man in him is completely gone, leaving behind only the all-comprehending sense of the divine. If an animal bites one of his arms, he is ready to give it his other arm also, and say that it is the Lord's will. Everything that comes to him is from the Lord. He does not show himself to men, and yet he is a magazine of love and of true and sweet ideas.

Next in order come the men with more Rajas or activity, combative natures who take up the ideas of the perfect ones and preach them to the world. The highest kind of men silently collect true and noble ideas, and others—the Buddhas and Christs—go from place to place preaching them and working for them. In the life of Gautama Buddha we notice him constantly saying that he is the twenty-fifth Buddha. The twenty-four before him are unknown to history, although the Buddha known to history must have built upon foundations laid by them. The highest men are calm, silent, and unknown. They are the men who really know the power of thought; they are sure that, even if they go into a cave and close the door and simply think five true thoughts and then pass away, these five thoughts of theirs will live through eternity. Indeed such thoughts will penetrate through the mountains, cross the oceans, and travel through the world. They will enter deep into human hearts and brains and raise up men and women

who will give them practical expression in the
workings of human life. These Sattvika men are
too near the Lord to be active and to fight, to
be working, struggling, preaching, and doing
good, as they say, here on earth to humanity.
The active workers, however good, have still a
little remnant of ignorance left in them. When
our nature has yet some impurities left in it, then
alone can we work. It is in the nature of work
to be impelled ordinarily by motive and by
attachment. In the presence of an ever-active
Providence who notes even the sparrow's fall,
how can man attach any importance to his own
work? Will it not be a blasphemy to do so when
we know that He is taking care of the minutest
things in the world? We have only to stand in
awe and reverence before Him saying, "Thy will
be done". The highest men cannot work, for in
them there is no attachment. Those whose whole
soul is gone into the Self, those whose desires
are confined in the Self, who have become ever
associated with the Self, for them there is no
work. Such are indeed the highest of mankind;
but apart from them everyone else has to work.
In so working we should never think that we
can help on even the least thing in this universe.
We cannot. We only help ourselves in this
gymnasium of the world. This is the proper
attitude of work. If we work in this way, if we

always remember that our present opportunity to work thus is a privilege which has been given to us, we shall never be attached to anything. Millions like you and me think that we are great people in the world; but we all die, and in five minutes the world forgets us. But the life of God is infinite. "Who can live a moment, breathe a moment, if this all-powerful One does not will it?" He is the ever-active Providence. All power is His and within His command. Through His command the winds blow, the sun shines, the earth lives, and death stalks upon the earth. He is the all in all; He is all and in all. We can only worship Him. Give up all fruits of work; do good for its own sake; then alone will come perfect non-attachment. The bonds of the heart will thus break, and we shall reap perfect freedom. This freedom is indeed the goal of Karma-Yoga.

THE IDEAL OF KARMA-YOGA

THE grandest idea in the religion of the Vedanta is that we may reach the same goal by different paths; and these paths I have generalised into four—viz those of work, love, psychology, and knowledge. But you must, at the same time, remember that these divisions are not very marked and quite exclusive of each other. Each blends into the other. But according to the type which prevails, we name the divisions. It is not that you can find men who have no other faculty than that of work, nor that you can find men who are no more than devoted worshippers only, nor that there are men who have no more than mere knowledge. These divisions are made in accordance with the type or the tendency that may be seen to prevail in a man. We have found that, in the end, all these four paths converge and become one. All religions and all methods of work and worship lead us to one and the same goal.

I have already tried to point out that goal. It is freedom as I understand it. Everything that we perceive around us is struggling towards freedom, from the atom to the man, from the insentient, lifeless particle of matter to the highest existence on earth, the human soul. The whole universe is in fact the result of this struggle for freedom. In all combinations every particle is trying to go on its own way, to fly from the other particles; but the others are holding it in check. Our earth is trying to fly away from the sun, and the moon from the earth. Everything has a tendency to infinite dispersion. All that we see in the universe has for its basis this one struggle towards freedom; it is under the impulse of this tendency that the saint prays and the robber robs. When the line of action taken is not a proper one, we call it evil; and when the manifestation of it is proper and high, we call it good. But the impulse is the same, the struggle towards freedom. The saint is oppressed with the knowledge of his condition of bondage, and he wants to get rid of it; so he worships God. The thief is oppressed with the idea that he does not possess certain things, and he tries to get rid of that want, to obtain freedom from it; so he steals. Freedom is the one goal of all nature, sentient or insentient; and, consciously or unconsciously, everything is struggling towards that goal. The freedom which the saint seeks is very different from that which the robber seeks; the freedom loved by the saint leads him to the enjoyment of infinite, unspeakable bliss, while that on which the robber has set his heart only forges other bonds for his soul.

There is to be found in every religion the manifestation of this struggle towards freedom. It is the groundwork of all morality, of unselfishness, which means getting rid of the idea that men are the same as their little body. When we see a man doing good work, helping others, it means that he cannot be confined within the limited circle of "me and mine". There is no limit to this getting out of selfishness. All the great systems of ethics preach absolute unselfishness as the goal. Supposing this absolute unselfishness can be reached by a man, what becomes of him? He is no more the little Mr. So-and-so; he has acquired infinite expansion. That little personality which he had before is now lost to him for ever; he has become infinite, and the attainment of this infinite expansion is indeed the goal of all religions and of all moral and philosophical teachings. The personalist, when he hears this idea philosophically put, gets frightened. At the same time, if he preaches morality, he after all teaches the very same idea himself. He puts no limit to the unselfishness of man. Suppose a man becomes perfectly unselfish under the personalistic system, how are we to distinguish him from the perfected ones in other systems? He has become one with the universe and to become that is the goal of all; only the poor personalist has not the courage to follow

out his own reasoning to its right conclusion.
Karma-Yoga is the attaining through unselfish
work of that freedom which is the goal of all
human nature. Every selfish action, therefore,
retards our reaching the goal, and every unselfish
action takes us towards the goal; that is why the
only definition that can be given of morality is
this: *That which is selfish is immoral, and that
which is unselfish is moral.*

But if you come to details, the matter will not
be seen to be quite so simple. For instance,
environment often makes the details different as
I have already mentioned. The same action
under one set of circumstances may be unselfish,
and under another set quite selfish. So we can
give only a general definition, and leave the
details to be worked out by taking into consideration the differences in time, place, and circumstances. In one country one kind of conduct
is considered moral, and in another the very
same is immoral, because the circumstances
differ. The goal of all nature is freedom, and
freedom is to be attained only by perfect unselfishness; every thought, word, or deed that is
unselfish takes us towards the goal and, as such,
is called moral. That definition, you will find,
holds good in every religion and every system of
ethics. In some systems of thought morality is
derived from a Superior Being—God. If you ask

why a man ought to do this and not that, their
answer is: "Because such is the command of
God." But whatever be the source from which it
is derived, their code of ethics also has the same
central idea—not to think of self but to give up
self. And yet some persons, in spite of this high
ethical idea, are frightened at the thought of
having to give up their little personalities. We
may ask the man who clings to the idea of little
personalities to consider the case of a person
who has become perfectly unselfish, who has no
thought for himself, who does no deed for him
self, who speaks no word for himself, and then
say where his "himself" is. That "himself" is
known to him only so long as he thinks, acts,
or speaks for himself. If he is only conscious of
others, of the universe, and of the all, where is
his "himself"? It is gone for ever.

Karma-Yoga, therefore, is a system of ethics
and religion intended to attain freedom through
unselfishness and by good works. The Karma-
Yogi need not believe in any doctrine whatever.
He may not believe even in God, may not ask
what his soul is, nor think of any metaphysical
speculation. He has got his own special aim of
realising selflessness; and he has to work it out
himself. Every moment of his life must be realisation, because he has to solve by mere work,
without the help of doctrine or theory, the very

same problem to which the Jnâni applies his reason and inspiration and the Bhakta his love.

Now comes the next question: What is this work? What is this doing good to the world? Can we do good to the world? In an absolute sense, no; in a relative sense, yes. No permanent or everlasting good can be done to the world; if it could be done, the world would not be this world. We may satisfy the hunger of a man for five minutes, but he will be hungry again. Every pleasure with which we supply a man may be seen to be momentary. No one can permanently cure this ever-recurring fever of pleasure and pain. Can any permanent happiness be given to the world? In the ocean we cannot raise a wave without causing a hollow somewhere else. The sum total of the good things in the world has been the same throughout in its relation to man's need and greed. It cannot be increased or decreased. Take the history of the human race as we know today. Do we not find the same miseries and the same happiness, the same pleasures and pains, the same differences in position? Are not some rich, some poor, some high, some low, some healthy, some unhealthy? All this was just the same with the Egyptians, the Greeks, and the Romans in ancient times as it is with the Americans today. So far as history is known, it has always been the same; yet at

the same time we find that running along with
all these incurable differences of pleasure and
pain, there has ever been the struggle to allevi-
ate them. Every period of history has given birth
to thousands of men and women who have
worked hard to smooth the passage of life for
others. And how far have they succeeded? We
can only play at driving the ball from one place
to another. We take away pain from the physical
plane, and it goes to the mental one. It is like
that picture in Dante's hell where the misers
were given a mass of gold to roll up a hill. Every
time they rolled it up a little, it again rolled
down. All our talks about the millennium are
very nice as schoolboy's stories, but they are no
better than that. All nations that dream of the
millennium also think that, of all peoples in the
world, they will have the best of it then for
themselves. This is the wonderfully unselfish
idea of the millennium!

We cannot add happiness to this world; similarly we cannot add pain to it either. The sum
total of the energies of pleasure and pain dis-
played here on earth will be the same throughout. We just push it from this side to the other
side, and from that side to this; but it will remain the same, because to remain so is its very
nature. This ebb and flow, this rising and falling,
is in the world's very nature; it would be as

logical to hold otherwise as to say that we may have life without death. This is complete nonsense, because the very idea of life implies death, and the very idea of pleasure implies pain. The lamp is constantly burning out, and that is its life. If you want to have life, you have to die every moment for it. Life and death are only different expressions of the same thing looked at from different standpoints; they are the falling and rising of the same wave, and the two form one whole. One looks at the "fall" side and becomes a pessimist, another looks at the "rise" side and becomes an optimist. When a boy is going to school and his father and mother are takng care of him, everything seems blessed to him; his wants are simple, he is a great optimist. But the old man, with his varied experience, becomes calmer and is sure to have his warmth considerably cooled down. So old nations, with signs of decay all around them, are apt to be less hopeful than new nations. There is a proverb in India, "A thousand years a city, and a thousand years a forest." This change of city into forest and vice versa is going on everywhere, and it makes people optimists or pessimists according to the side they see of it.

The next idea we take up is the idea of equality. These millennium ideas have been great

motive powers to work. Many religions preach
this as an element in them—that God is coming
to rule the universe, and that then there will be
no difference at all in conditions. The people
who preach this doctrine are mere fanatics, and
fanatics are indeed the sincerest of mankind.
Christianity was preached just on the basis of
the fascination of this fanaticism, and that is
what made it so attractive to the Greek and the
Roman slaves. They believed that under the
millennial religion there would be no more
slavery, that there would be plenty to eat and
drink; and therefore they flocked round the
Christian standard. Those who preached the idea
first were of course ignorant fanatics, but very
sincere. In modern times this millennial aspira-
tion takes the form of equality—of liberty,
equality, and fraternity. This is also fanaticism.
True equality has never been and never can be
on earth. How can we all be equal here? This
impossible kind of equality implies total death.
What makes this world what it is? Lost balance.
In the primal state, which is called chaos, there
is perfect balance. How do all the formative
forces of the universe come then? By struggling,
competition, conflict. Suppose that all the particles of matter were held in equilibrium, would
there be then any process of creation? We know
from science that it is impossible. Disturb a

sheet of water, and there you find every particle of the water trying to become calm again, one rushing against the other; and in the same way all the phenomena which we call the universe— all things therein—are struggling to get back to the state of perfect balance. Again a disturbance comes, and again we have combination and creation. Inequality is the very basis of creation. At the same time the forces struggling to obtain equality are as much a necessity of creation as those which destroy it.

Absolute equality, that which means a perfect balance of all the struggling forces in all the planes, can never be in this world. Before you attain that state, the world will have become quite unfit for any kind of life, and no one will be there. We find, therefore, that all these ideas of the millennium and of absolute equality are not only impossible but also that, if we try to carry them out, they will lead us surely enough to the day of destruction. What makes the difference between man and man? It is largely the difference in the brain. Nowadays no one but a lunatic will say that we are all born with the same brain power. We come into the world with unequal endowments; we come as greater men or as lesser men, and there is no getting away from that pre-natally determined condition. The American Indians were in this country for thousands of years, and a few handfuls of your ancestors came to their land. What difference have they caused in the appearance of the country! Why did not the Indians make improvements and build cities, if all were equal? With your ancestors a different sort of brain power came into the land, different bundles of past impressions came, and they worked out and manifested themselves. Absolute non-differentiation is death. So long as this world lasts, differentiation there will and must be, and the millennium of perfect equality will come only when a cycle of creation comes to its end. Before that, equality cannot be. Yet this idea of realising the millennium is a great motive power. Just as inequality is necessary for creation itself. so the struggle to limit it is also necessary. If there were no struggle to become free and get back to God, there would be no creation either. It is the difference between these two forces that determines the nature of the motives of men. There will always be these motives to work, some tending towards bondage and others towards freedom.

This world's wheel within wheel is a terrible mechanism; if we put our hands in it, as soon as we are caught we are gone. We all think that when we have done a certain duty, we shall be at rest; but before we have done a part of that duty, another is already in waiting. We are all being dragged along by this mighty, complex world-machine. There are only two ways out of it; one is to give up all concern with the machine, to let it go and stand aside, to give up our desires. That is very easy to say, but is almost impossible to do. I do not know whether in twenty millions of men one can do that. The other way is to plunge into the world and learn the secret of work, and that is the way of Karma-Yoga. Do not fly away from the wheels of the world-machine, but stand inside it and learn the secret of work. Through proper work done inside, it is also possible to come out. Through this machinery itself is the way out.

We have now seen what work is. It is a part of nature's foundation and goes on always. Those that believe in God understand this better, because they know that God is not such an incapable being as will need our help. Although this universe will go on always, our goal is freedom, our goal is unselfishness; and according to Karma-Yoga, that goal is to be reached through work. All ideas of making the world perfectly happy may be good as motive powers for fanatics; but we must know that fanaticism brings forth as much evil as good. The Karma-Yogi asks why you require any motive to work other than the inborn love of freedom. Be beyond the common worldly motives. "To work you have the right, but not to the fruits thereof." Man can train himself to know and to practise that, says the Karma-Yogi. When the idea of doing good becomes a part of his very being, then he will not seek for any motive outside. Let us do good because it is good to do good; he who does good work even in order to get to heaven binds himself down, says the Karma-Yogi. Any work that is done with any the least selfish motive, instead of making us free, forges one more chain for our feet.

So the only way is to give up all the fruits of work, to be unattached to them. Know that this world is not we, nor are we this world; that we are really not the body; that we really do not work. We are the Self, eternally at rest and at peace. Why should we be bound by anything? It is very good to say that we should be perfectly non-attached, but what is the way to do it? Every good work we do without any ulterior motive, instead of forging a new chain, will break one of the links in the existing chains. Every good thought that we send to the world without thinking of any return, will be stored up there and break one link in the chain and make us purer and purer, until we become the purest of mortals. Yet all this may seem to be rather quixotic and too philosophical, more theoretical than practical. I have read many arguments against the Bhagavad-Gita, and many have said that without motives you cannot work. They have never seen unselfish work except under the influence of fanaticism, and therefore they speak in that way.

Let me tell you in conclusion a few words about one man who actually carried this teaching of Karma-Yoga into practice. That man is Buddha. He is the one man who ever carried this into perfect practice. All the prophets of the world, except Buddha, had external motives to move them to unselfish action. The prophets of the world, with this single exception, may be divided into two sets—one set holding that they are incarnations of God come down on earth, and the other holding that they are only messengers from God; and both draw their impetus for work from outside, expect reward from outside, however highly spiritual may be the language they use. But Buddha is the only prophet who said, "I do not care to know your various theories about God. What is the use of discussing all the subtle doctrines about the soul? Do good and be good. And this will take you to freedom and to whatever truth there is." He was, in the conduct of his life, absolutely without personal motives; and what man worked more than he? Show me in history one character who has soared so high above all. The whole human race has produced but one such character, such high philosophy, such wide sympathy. This great philosopher, preaching the highest philosophy, yet has the deepest sympathy for the lowest of animals, and never puts forth any claims for himself. He is the ideal Karma-Yogi, acting entirely without motive, and the history of humanity shows him to have been the greatest man ever born; beyond compare the greatest combination of heart and brain that ever existed, the greatest soul-power that has ever been manifested. He is the first great reformer the world has seen. He is the first who dared to say, "Believe not because some old manuscripts are produced, believe not because it is your national belief, because you have been made to believe it from your childhood; but reason it all out, and after you have analysed it, then, if you find that it will do good to one and all, believe it, live up to it, and help others to live up to it." He works best who works without any motive, neither for money, nor for fame, nor for anything else; and when a man can do that, he will be a Buddha, and out of him will come the power to work in such a manner as will transform the world. This man represents the very highest ideal of Karma-Yoga.